a HOME AT last

A HOUSING PROGRAM FOR THE MENTALLY ILL

EMILY RUSH ○ JASON HALBUER ○ NOAH HOPCHIN

Edited by Bianca Ho

Golden Meteorite Press

Edmonton Alberta Canada

Designed and edited by Bianca Ho

Published by Golden Meteorite Press.

126 Kingsway Garden
Post Office Box 34181
Edmonton, Alberta, Canada T5G 3G4
Telephone: 1-(780)-378-0063
Email: aamardon@yahoo.ca
Website: www.austinmardon.org

Library and Archives Canada Cataloguing in Publication
Rush, Emily, 1981-
[Room for change]
          A home at last : a housing program for the mentally ill / Emily Rush,
Jason Halbauer, Noah Hopchin, Bianca Ho.

Revision of: Room for change.
Includes bibliographical references.
ISBN 978-1-897472-83-5 (pbk.)

          1. Homelessness--Alberta. 2. Shelters for the homeless--Alberta.
3. Champion's Centre. 4. Mentally ill--Housing--Alberta. 5. Mental health
services--Alberta. I. Halbauer, Jason, 1984-, author II. Hopchin, Noah,
1983-, author III. Ho, Bianca, author IV. Title. V. Title: Room for change.

HD7287.96.C32A42 2013   363.5'1575097123   C2013-905542-8

TABLE OF CONTENTS

"the **most** POVERTY TERRIBLE

is LONELINESS

and the *feeling*

OF BEING

UNLOVED."

— MOTHER TERESA

INTRO

We are three college students. Noah and Jason were hired by The Champion's Centre through the Government of Canada's Summer Career Placement Grant, but I volunteered. Together, we spent the summer of 2006 writing this book. It was an excellent opportunity for us to gain valuable work experience and insight into the social issues surrounding The Champion's Centre.

Circumstance can play a large role. Many people who find themselves without homes also suffer from mental illnesses. Victims of mental illnesses are unlikely to make logical or rational choices. Mental illnesses take away a person's ability to lead a productive and heathy life.

The homeless do not necessarily suffer from laziness—they are need of assistance to get back on track. Berating or shouting demeaning comments at a homeless person will not help him or her. Such behaviour will only demonstrate the ignorance of the problems that many homeless people face and deal with. They seek recognition and acknowledgement from others; they want to be treated like regular human beings.

During our time at The Champion's Centre's Ponoka facility, we had a chance to meet many of the tenants. We had expected the centre to be hectic, but it was actually quite comfortable. It did not take long for our expectations to be proven wrong.

It was almost time for dinner when we arrived, Fred Klooster, the centre's manager in Ponoka, invited us in and sat us down. A few of the tenants were talking and joking around, others were sitting peacefully as they waited for dinner. After everyone said grace, dinner was served. Some ate quicker than others, but it felt comfortable and it was just like dinner at home. Though we didn't speak our thoughts at the time, I think we were all surprised with the atmosphere. Some of the tenants asked Margaret, the server for seconds, and others thanked her for cleaning their plates. Everyone was polite and it was a pleasant atmosphere.

Later on that evening we had an opportunity to talk with some of the centre's tenants. Even though not all of them wanted to be interviewed, they were all very friendly. We're grateful they were kind enough to share their home with us for the night. We learned a lot during our stay.

It was interesting to learn about where and how The Champion's Centre started and be physically there to experience and see the progress that has been made since. We were able understand the centre as a concept rather than a facility that provided types of housing options. We hope that you will enjoy reading about The Champion's Centre.

– Emily Rush

"POVERTY is a NOOSE THAT STRANGLES humility & breeds DISRESPECT for God+MAN."

—AMERICAN INDIAN PROVERB

EMILY

On a chilly autumn day, I was waiting for my bus at the terminal. I sat down on the benches outside the heated waiting area. I occasionally glanced at my watch and looked at the people milling around the bus station. It was quite busy for a Tuesday afternoon; some people were waiting on benches nearby and others were standing on the opposite side of the glass partition from me. It was nearly five o'clock in the evening and many of the people had probably finished work and were headed home. School had ended earlier, so there weren't many youths.

Out of the corner of my eye, I noticed a Native man looking in a nearby garbage can. He walked past me, picked up an abandoned coffee cup on the bench across from me and sat down.

"There's some left in here, and it's still kinda warm," he said to me with a smile. This man was scruffy and dirty, the typical homeless man that I wouldn't usually have a conversation with, but he seemed kind. I returned the smile as he sat down beside me and sipped his found coffee.

He noticed the few textbooks and notebooks on my lap and asked me about them. I explained that I had just finished class at a school nearby and was about to head home.

"I never went to school," he began. "I needed to make some money, so I started working construction up in Grande Prairie. I did that for a long time, but I got a lead on a job down here in Edmonton. I packed my DEQ and hopped on the bus. I got here and there was no job for me. I had no money or place to stay. I didn't know anyone around here either," he explained to me as he stared at the ground.

I glanced at the people around me to see if anyone was listening to us chat. There were a few people around, but no one was looking in our direction. Perhaps someone might assume he was intoxicated? But it was very clear when he spoke to me, he was sober.

"Did you try searching for another job? Could your family send you money to get home?" I asked him quietly.

He told me his family was poor and that he had given up his apartment when he moved down here. "I dunno what to do. I try to stay at the shelters, but they're usually full," he said.

"I don't get down about what's happened to me. I know that this too is in God's plan. All I can do is pray about it. Even if it isn't clear to me right now, it will be someday."

He smiled again and took another sip of his coffee.

It was astonishing to hear his steadfast faith, considering his situation. What struck me about him was his positive, hopeful attitude. I wondered how many people out there had stories similar to his, but gave in to the desperation and turned to drugs and alcohol to pull through each day.

"I remember the day that I found God. It's a kinda crazy story, but I was searching through a dumpster in the alley behind a restaurant near here when it happened. Anyway, I looked up and I felt like I was in a haze and a voice spoke to me... deep inside. I just knew that things were out of my hands and there was a higher power watching over me."

Some people have a hard time talking about their beliefs, but he was very open about his. He told me that he was just so grateful to be saved, that he would gladly share his story with anyone who would listen. As

I listened, I thought about my experiences with religion. I consider myself a spiritual person, but merely calling myself "spiritual" seemed to lack the commitment that many Christians have made to their faith. I felt embarrassed about my inability to connect with him.

The man didn't seem to notice that I was deep in thought and moved onto another topic. He was chatting about his former life and self. "I miss my old home and the stuff I used to do everyday, but what I miss most from my old life is my art. I used to do some carving and I really liked it. I mostly carved soapstone and stuff... Anyway, it was nice to have something to work on all the time."

He played with the coffee cup lid and let his eyes close a little. "I used to love to sing too. I knew lots of songs and would sing all the time to my daughter." He lowered his head a little and was still.

After a moment or two, he began singing a haunting native song that was hardly a whisper with all the noise of the bus station. His voice was faint and wavered at times.

Looking up, I noticed the bus was making its way around the curb, heading into the terminal area and I saw a few men looking over at me, trying to get my attention. I knew instinctively they were concerned that this homeless man was harassing me. They wanted to step in and save me from the penniless man. I felt anger welling up inside my chest. This man wasn't doing anything wrong. I wanted let everyone know that he hadn't harassed me for money at all. Instead, I fiddled with my books and looked at the ground.

These guys were willing to look out for me, a white middle-class girl, but what about everyone else? What about the homeless man? What are they doing for him besides assuming that he is going to hurt or annoy me? They don't know his past. They don't know that he once had a job similar to theirs.

I stood up and handed the homeless man a five-dollar bill. "Here, go get yourself a hot cup of coffee," I said smiling. "It was a pleasure to meet you and you have given me a lot to think about."

He smiled up at me and grasped my hand in his.

"You are truly an angel. I am very lucky to have someone like you as a friend," he said as he shook my hand. Walking to my bus. I shifted my textbooks in my hands. They felt heavy and awkward. I stared out the bus window and thought about the person I had just met.

That homeless man is a human being. He has fallen on hard times, but was a more humble, decent person than any that discriminator.

I would be lying if I said that my social conditioning had not needled paranoid thoughts in at the back of my mind. What if he hangs out there waiting for me everyday because I gave him money and he expects more? What if he follows me home? Was talking to him a good idea?

Each doubtful thought blew to pieces as I recalled his hopeful eyes and the way he grasped my hand and shook it, calling me his friend. It wouldn't be such a bad thing to run into a nice person like him once in a while. The experience that day opened my eyes to the reality of homelessness—not every homeless person is an addict, not every homeless person asks for money from a passer-by. In reality, I doubted I would ever see him again. But from then on, I promised myself to try to look each homeless person in the eye and see beyond the surface.

"if a *free* SOCIETY cannot HELP the **MANY** who are POOR, IT cannot SAVE *the* FEW WHO are Rich."

—JOHN FITZGERALD KENNEDY

NOAH

These days, I don't find myself on Edmonton's Whyte Avenue as often as I once did. Whyte Avenue is a cultural nexus in Edmonton. It's close to the University of Alberta and just across the river from the downtown core. It's packed with bars and nightclubs, upscale and shabby hotels, a variety of restaurants, head shops, and boutique clothing stores. Although the area tries hard to maintain a trendy visage, it's also one of the places in Edmonton where the city's homelessness crisis is most visible.

Regrettably, I have dealt with the problem of homelessness on Whyte Avenue the same way I have seen most people do. I walk at a pace much brisker than my normal pace, so that homeless people are less likely to approach me for change. My gazes constantly wanders around in an effort to appear as though I am scanning the streetscape. When I am, in fact, carefully trying to keep the homeless in my peripheral vision so I can avoid making accidental direct eye contact with them. When I think about it, I'm amazed by the number of times I've been 'fascinated' by an empty lot.

Despite my best efforts, I am inevitably asked for money. The excuse of not have cash on me, "Sorry, I only have debit", is a response I find myself giving fairly often. Most of the time I say it earnestly, though

I'm certain I have delivered it as a hasty excuse as I continued my brisk pace, with change jingling in my pockets. But more often than not, if I'm asked for change and I have it, I give it away. I do it reluctantly, not because I feel a particular attachment to the money I am giving away. If I returned from a walk down Whyte Avenue to find that all of my coins had fallen through a hole in my pocket, I wouldn't be terribly upset. I am disappointed when I give away coins. People ask me for change, but all I can bring myself to give them is a few lousy coins.

I have had firsthand experience with a mental illness. It was considerably mild, but it has given me some insight into the issue of homelessness. I suffered from depression for a period of time. I went through days where I could not tell the difference between not wanting to do anything and not being able to do anything. I had assumed it was the former, and that perhaps I was being lazy. I assumed all I needed to do was just change my attitude to rectify the situation. I suppose attitude is a part of it, but it is much easier said than done.

Mental illness is one of the major causes of homelessness. It's difficult to acknowledge the reality of many homeless individuals not having the proper support networks to provide aid and encouragement. Most of these people blame themselves for their illness—it's heartbreaking. They blame themselves for being different, for being unable to hold down a job, for being unable to communicate properly, and for being unable to support themselves. They feel guilty for letting people in their lives down.

Homes need support; people need support. I was fortunate to have a fantastic and understanding support network that has made possible for me hold my ground. I felt guilty for letting others down when I was dealing with depression. I received help and had a support network that allowed me to deal with my condition and continue to persevere when I could have easily been in a situation without a support network. I could have been in a situation with people blaming me for factors beyond my control. I was fortunate, but I know many aren't.

Mental illness can be an intangible sickness. In some cases, others can observe how a mental illness manifests itself within an individual's behaviour. It doesn't always paint a complete picture of how the individual is affected by his or her illness. Once, while purchasing a copy of the street newspaper, *Our Voice*, from a homeless man, I saw that he had a lot of difficulty with speaking. Just from observing I could not tell whether he had difficulty forming complete thoughts or if it was a problem expressing his thoughts. Perhaps he was able to think clearly, but could not coherently express those thoughts because his brain was not in proper control of his body.

Almost anyone can observe the symptoms of severe mental illness, but problems often arise when the presence of a mental illness is less apparent. To the untrained observer, it appears as if there is no problem. Unlike many illnesses, we, as individuals and as a society, have trouble observing the effects of mental illness.

It has been my experience that mental illnesses, even depression, is grossly misunderstood by the public at large. Even though I have experience with depression, I cannot pretend to fully understand. In fact, it took me years to even come to accept and understand that it does have an effect on me. I think the problem is that none of us really see what mental illness does to us. It isn't like any of the illness we are traditionally used to dealing with. It is possible to observe how cancerous cells attack specific organs and move to others, destroying them as they go. It is possible to observe how leprosy erodes and destroys the nervous system and the physical appearance of flesh. We see the physical damage. Mental illnesses don't have a physical form. Even though it affects the brain, it doesn't physically destroy it the way most illnesses destroy their target organs. Mental illness is an acid that slowly corrodes the mind. It leads to shatter the lifestyle that the victims know of— the connections in our lives: our relationships, our sense of self, our sense of belonging, and our homes. Often, the victims are accused, people they have relationships and connections with blame the victims for having failed to properly maintain their lives. Mental illnesses in many cases, take away and detract from a person's relationships, which is support system they need.

The Champion's Centre is an organization that strives to provide a support network. It offers stability to the unstable. It helps people hold the connections in place while these victims reinforce them.

"HOW does it FEEL to be WITHOUT a home? just like A COMPLETE unknown like A Rolling stone."

—BOB DYLAN

JASON

Homeless people have asked us for help, there is no denying it. Many times when you walk by a homeless person, they ask for help. They may have a hat sitting in front of them. They may do their best to get our attention as we stroll on by with everything on our minds but them. They may even try to stop us and state their case—trying tell us how they're just like us. But, we don't want to hear it.

We often believe that these people somehow brought homelessness upon themselves through the choices they made in their lives. We don't think that they're worthy of our attention. We prefer to believe that they're drug addicts, drunks, and deadbeat more often than a more likely reality; victims of circumstance. It's easier not to treat them as people; it's easier blow right by them without acknowledgement. They're strangers. You won't be meeting them again at a social gathering. They are easy to forget.

I've seen homeless people be refused simple requests. Things as simple as asking for the time. They are treated rudely, or even ignored.

Long ago, I was in a café, when I saw a homeless person walk in and ask for a cup of water. He even offered to pay for it. He was scrawny and there were four people working there at the time. The lady at the counter couldn't possibly ignore him, so she went and grabbed the manager. The manager granted him his request on the condition that he would drink it quickly and leave. It would be understandable if there was a barrage of homeless people in the store that could possible disrupt the business. Why can't a skinny, non-threatening man sit down for a minute and have a drink of water? If we aren't ignoring them or mistreating them, we use compromising methods to deal them.

I have seen one homeless person in St. Albert, a rich suburbia north of Edmonton, and everybody knows him by name. But, we don't know his story. I've lived in St. Albert my entire life. We don't have to think about how to deal with the homeless; out of sight, out of mind. We have no reason to feel sympathy.

We give ourselves excuses to ignore the homeless, so we can go on with our lives. Sometimes, there are even anecdotes: "I've heard that he's actually a millionaire and he spends half of his year in Mexico-and the other half on the street. I've also heard that he is a scientist doing research about street-life. I'm curious why this type of experiment would take over ten years." I'm not sure where these stories came from, but I do know that they take a load off our minds. I've heard other myths about the homeless, too. "They have a house. They're just scamming you." Somehow, I just don't believe that people are out on the streets in the cold to seam a couple of dollars off of the generous. And then there is my favourite: "They make more in a day begging than we do going to work. They could easily afford a place." That isn't true. They don't make enough. Without enough money to afford a home, it complicates matters. It's almost impossible to hold a job without legal residence. We try as hard as we can to justify our unjust actions; to wrong the rights in our mind. These justifications are just too fallible.

Our beliefs are erratic. We are selective in what we want to believe. Perhaps if I were to keep buying a lottery ticket every day, I could win. But what are the chances? The odds of winning the Lotto 6/49 are roughly 1 in 13 841 287 201. Despite the minute odds, it doesn't stop people from buying lottery tickets, the hope is still there. We would rather believe that we would be more likely to win the lottery than for us to end up homeless. One out of six children is living below the poverty line (*Campaign* 2000, 2006). That means one child out of six is on the verge of homelessness. It is a scary thing to think about. It's a terrible life. But you're probably somewhere warm surrounded by loved ones. It could never happen to you, right?

It's just a matter of your support system breaking down. As of right now, you may have a job, a family, and friends. What if you lose your job? What if your close family passes away? What if you move? Or maybe your friends just aren't in a position to help you.

Does it still seem unlikely? Well, think of how many people are possibly less fortunate than you. Maybe these people don't have family to support them. They may have more serious problems; they may be financial, emotional, physical or mental barriers. The truth is, we are so self-absorbed that we don't want to think about their problems. I use the 'we' instead of 'you' because I don't exclude myself from this equation. I don't want to constantly accuse, I am just as guilty. At one point in my life, I ignored the plight of homeless people. If I wasn't ignoring them, I would have assumed they deserved it or that it wasn't as bad as it seemed. No good person could be in such a bad circumstance, right?

I recall being approached by a homeless lady. When she came closer, I saw that she had very few teeth and she had the stench of vomit. She asked me if I had a second, when I told her that I did, she told me her story. She spoke of how her alcoholism had taken over her life. She was on the street before she knew it.

I tried to put myself in her shoes. I tried to imagine forcing myself up, freezing cold and hungry, out from inside the dumpster that I used to salvage some warmth. I tried to imagine begging for everything I needed. I tried to imagine people scorning me and ignoring me as it I blended into the streetscape; I became a street lamp, a sewer drain even. Some people acknowledge me as a person, but it's not the kind of friendly chat I'm looking for. An important-looking man in a business suit perhaps, or maybe it's a girl with shopping bags who tells me how worthless I am: "Go get a job, you bum." I couldn't just walk into an office building and ask for a job without nice clothes or a shower. It's not even possible to get a job without a permanent residence. No job I could get would provide me with enough income have a residence. I tried to imagine the sting of such accusations, tried to imagine getting used to living below everything, getting used to not being human. As she described further, I tried to imagine my life as a system of cause and effect. I'm hungry, I panhandle to buy food, I drink to forget or to pass the time. I'm tired, so I sleep. The only reason I do anything is because I am living out of habit.

I tried to imagine it all, but I couldn't. At the end of the story, I was still meeting a friend for lunch in a warm restaurant. I still lived with my parents and I knew I was going to be sleeping indoors for the night.

After being pushed down by so many people and things, she was able to smile. I was amazed she was able to look me in the eyes and smile as warmly as she did. She told me I reminded her of someone she used to know, someone who offered her a place to stay. She told me she rejected the home because she was an alcoholic and she knew she would cause problems. Her story had only lasted for five minutes, but after she had finished, I didn't know what to say.

I was touched. In my youth and ignorance, I had thought that she wanted money. I didn't have any, and I told her so without her asking me. She looked very disappointed. She didn't want my money. She very well might have needed it, but she didn't want it. She wanted someone to treat her like a human being, an equal. She wanted me to realize that she was as made of flesh and blood, just as I am. She wanted to relate to me. More importantly, she wanted then what I want now; she wanted to educate the public.

If the public learn to understand homeless people, they will take steps to help. The public will see them as people with problems, rather than simply homeless. Homeless people have problems. That isn't a surprise to anyone. They are characterized by a lack of a home. They are grouped with the jobless, useless, and hopeless.

The way we refer to homeless people is an issue. What if I referred to everyone I know by what they lack? "Hey, there goes motherless Dave", or "This is my friend, jobless Susan." The word 'homeless is often used as a noun, not an adjective. 'Homeless is a term that has been normalized. They have become things, we don't refer to them as people; they have become objects. They are unpleasant sights. They are things that interrupt our day. The word 'homeless' is meant to be an adjective, a descriptive word for person or people. We focus on what they don't have. Whether we refer to them as 'homeless people' or 'the homeless, the use of either of the terms has an underlying denotation of what they lack. We are choosing to not acknowledge that they are also human beings that have feelings.

Why can't we just refer to them as 'people'? They are people living on the streets. They are people who are unable to care for themselves. They are people who can't turn their lives around without help.

The Champion's Centre offers help. It is a more effective system for dealing with the homelessness crisis. It is more feasible than group homes and more permanent. I was excited when I heard about them, and also why I wanted to be a part of this book. I think what Klaas Klooster and The Champion's Centre are doing for these people without homes is very important—they are putting people in need first.

"The STRENGTH of A nation DERIVES from THE integrity OF HOME."

—CONFUCIUS

MODEL

The Champion's Centre is run with Galatians 6:10 in mind: "Do good to everyone." This statement of charity reflects the centre's caring supportive attitude. Anyone in need is accepted as part of the centre's family and given the same benefits as everyone else. Everyone is equal and deserving of the same treatment and care; no one is ignored for what they look like, where they are from, or what they can or cannot do.

What are the options for a person facing eviction from his apartment or release from the Alberta Hospital in Ponoka? The Champion's Centre is a different take on traditional group homes. Where many group homes rely on government funding and large donations from the community, The Champion's Centre can also rely on the embedded businesses within its facilities. The concept for this type of group housing is that each centre is self-sustaining. The tenants pay rent each month and money made from the café and antiques store that each centre has goes directly into the operating costs and building upkeep. The antique stores that both the Ponoka centre and the Medicine Hat centre have are stocked with donations from Helping Hands Estate Services. They donate antique collectibles in exchange for a tax receipt. The tenants of the centres work in the Café or help out with the housekeeping if they are able to. It helps the tenants to socialize with the community, but eliminates the stress of a regular job.

Affordable housing is difficult to find. With a two percent vacancy rate in Edmonton and a zero percent vacancy rate in Red Deer and Calgary (*Housing Market Outlook*, 2006), it is no surprise that many people end up living on the street despite employment. Housing isn't possible for a person who works for minimum wage. The problem with homelessness continues to grow as the number of people moving to Alberta increases due to the economic boom.

Many people argue that there are many shelters, all with ample room for the homeless. Though there are shelters that can provide a warm place for a street person to go, many of the shelters turn away people because there isn't enough room. The shelters are also not equipped to give the support and medical help that some of the people require. There isn't much they can do for people with mental illnesses, other than give them a snack and let them warm up for a few hours."

Shelters are not the solution to homelessness—it is merely a temporary first aid solution for a much larger wound on our social structure, there needs to be a more permanent solution to actually solve the problem. Communities spend a lot of money to absorb the cost of a homeless person. The costs per month for the basic housing options an average homeless person has are staggering. There are costs for getting in trouble with the law, jail living costs, housing and care in psychiatric facilities, shelters. Many of the mentally ill need to be hospitalized and treated for their illnesses. Some of the people in psychiatric facilities could live outside the hospital with the proper guidance and support. According to Dr. Patrick White, President of the Alberta Psychiatric Association in a February 3rd, 2003 interview with the Edmonton Journal, "Part of the reason we're unable to discharge some of the people in to the community is because of [a] lack of housing."

It can be quite costly for a person with a disability to live on his or her own. Often times the only income that these unfortunate individuals have is the money from Assured Income for the Severely Handicapped or other pensions. With regular living expenses and medicine, it just isn't enough. "Most of a disability pension would go for the rent, let alone cable, utility, phone and groceries. The Champion's Centre offers a complete package for a reasonable price, which includes all of the above, along with linen changing and room cleaning once a week," says Klaas Klooster, Executive Director of the organization.

There are group homes available to those who are ready for transitional housing. This is a viable solution to the housing situation they may face upon leaving the hospital. Often, group homes can be costly and many are dependent government funding and/or community funding raised by non-profit organizations. If the government funding is pulled, the tenants face eviction from their homes. Group homes are only a temporary housing option for people who are mentally ill.

The Champion's Centre relies on interested people to contact the organization to open centres in communities with a need for supportive housing solutions. The organization takes a proactive approach in some communities as well, but they cannot reach everyone in need through touring and promotion alone.

If you are interested in bringing a centre to your community, there are steps that can be taken to begin the process. The Champion's Centre website, www.thechampionscentre.org, has request forms to open a centre. Using the contact information on the website, send the request form to Klaas, or contact him for more information about the centre and its concept. From there, you may need to create a local advisory board in your town to help with fundraising and locating a suitable building to house the facility. That way, in each step of the process there are people to help you, guide you and pray for your success in creating a Champion's Centre in your town. If you cannot invest the time and the energy into a project that large, you can still help The Champion's Centre by donating or volunteering with the organization.

Permanent supportive housing is a solution to the problem of homelessness among mentally people and those with developmental difficulties. This type of housing has the outreach support and services that people need to lead healthy lives. If centres are put in each community nationwide, the number of people facing life on the streets due to the lack of affordable housing will be greatly decreased.

"**NO ONE**
has **EVER** BECOME
POOR
by **GIVING**."

—ANNE FRANK

KLAAS KLOOSTER

Klaas is the Executive Director of The Champion's Centre. With the help many people, he has built the charity from the ground up with hard work and strong faith. Every day in his ministry and charitable work, he addresses problems our society faces. His personal history has a direct relevance to The Champion's Centre and its conception. Klaas' path has not been an easy one, but with the help of his family and God, he has come through trying situations and created a centre helping those in need.

Klaas grew up in Edmonton and was one of nine children in a Christian household. The Klooster family struggled to make ends meet, but their faith and perseverance pulled them through the difficult times. Religion was a large part of the family's routine; the children attended church service twice on Sundays; which includes Sunday school and catechism. With not much money left over for extracurricular activities, much of Klaas' time was spent with his family at home and at the church.

"Coming from such a large family, we were considered poor by the standards of those days," Klaas says. "My family was close and remains so. My brother, Fred, is the manager of the Ponoka Champion's Centre and was very instrumental, not so much in the renovations, but in planning and decorating to make it aesthetically pleasing. Other members of the family encouraged, prayed, and gave some financial support."

During his childhood, Klaas' father worked hard to sustain the family and their lifestyle. While juggling two jobs, the head of the Klooster family rarely had free time to spend with his family. Klaas missed his father and began working with him at his father's second job in a bakery on weekends. He worked Friday nights until six in the morning, running the bread machine to give his father a few hours of sleep.

Working became a priority for Klaas. He nearly failed ninth grade when was working full-time at the bakery. It was at the age of fourteen that Klaas first believed that God called him into ministry. For years afterwards, Klaas would struggle with the decision to become involved in God's work.

In eleventh grade, Klaas dropped out of high school to continue working full-time. His older siblings had been working for years, handing over paycheques to aid in supporting the household, until the time when they left—in some cases, moving out as young as age sixteen. During the trying times in the family's history this closeness and generosity was important to keep the household running, with food on the table and clothes on everyone's backs.

From time to time, Klaas became depressed and restless, constantly seeking new challenges. Throughout his adult years, his depression manifested itself in his dissatisfaction with different careers. Klaas believed that his depression was not caused by chemical imbalance, but that it was a spiritual one. He was still battling his calling to the church and was not sure he was ready to dedicate his life to God's work.

In his late teen years, Klaas met Joanne, the woman who would become his wife, while working at Van's Sausage Company. She is a year older and she worked part-time while she went to university. She was deeply involved with her church, and she met many of the friends through their weekly Bible study. As his family attended a different church than the one he grew up in, Klaas started to attend a church of a different denomination. Joanne invited him to join her at a Bible study one day, and shortly after he invited her to join him at his church.

"She was vibrant and full of life. It was then that I began to take notice of her," Klaas explains.

They became friends, but lost touch when he began working at another job. A few years later, the two happened upon each other at a grocery store. Klaas asked her out for coffee to catch up.

A year later, the two married. Klaas and Joanne have four children, two daughters and two sons. They had their first child, a girl, two years after they were married. In the subsequent year they had another girl, then a boy, and finally two years later, another boy. Klaas' children are now grown with children of their own.

For twenty years, Klaas worked in the grocery business, battling restlessness and depression that hid just beneath the surface. In 1998, Klaas received a Certificate in Ministry from Carey Theological College on the University of British Columbia campus. Klaas' interest and devotion to religious studies had been continuing throughout his adult life. After completing school, he was hired as a youth pastor and he was finally able to feel that his life was on the right track.

Almost two years into his youth pastorate, Klaas decided to resign his position at the church. He did not know it at the time, but he was in a severe clinical depression. He left his ministry work and concentrated on treating what he later learned was depression. For a year and a half, Klaas was deeply depressed—at times, he contemplated suicide.

Medication and faith were the keys to his recovery. The medication helped bring Klaas out of the worst of the depression, but it was while reading the Bible one day that he realized that, for him, depression was a choice, Klaas made a decision that day to commit his life to God. He found that he did not need medication any more and that his life had renewed his sense of purpose.

"For me it was a choice, but for others it might not be. I am not advocating that people try what I did," Klaas says. "Still, to this day, I consciously have to choose to be happy. I sometimes feel the depression coming on, but I reaffirm my trust in God and I can be happy in Him."

It is often in times of deep trouble and despair that people turn to God to guide them through. For Klaas, faith and devotion to God steered his life onto the right path; a path that would lead to the creation of The Champion's Centre.

After the haze of depression lifted from him, Klaas looked for a new business venture. Together with Joanne, they decided to search for a revenue property they could purchase. Klaas' brother, Fred, had recently retired at the time and was also looking for a new career. If they could find an apartment to buy, Fred could work as the caretaker.

At the time, Klaas had been working with a church youth worker from Hobbema. He noticed an abandoned restaurant nearby with an attached building that would be the perfect place to start an afterschool youth ministry and serve as a safe house for runaway teens. Klaas had the idea five years prior and had written it down if an opportunity ever presented itself. He did not pursue the idea due to a lack of support from the community and the church.

Over the next few years, the vision for the centre shifted away from the safe house idea. After noticing an unused medical building in Ponoka, Klaas and Joanne brainstormed for ways they could use the building. Because the Alberta Hospital is located in Ponoka, Klaas began researching group homes for mentally ill people and people with developmental disabilities. He discovered startling facts that changed the course of purpose for the centre.

Depression had touched his life, but he was able to recover and become strong enough to be in a position to help others. Some mentally ill people do not have the means to recover and support themselves. Klaas changed the intent of the centre to address a growing problem in Alberta and Canada.

"I was not aware of the problem of homelessness until I began researching it," he explains. "30 – 75 percent of homeless people have a mental illness. Not to mention that in many cases, these individuals, as a result of the illness, had burned all their bridges behind them."

The form that The Champion's Centre has taken on today was not his initial vision, but he feels that the centre took on the shape that it did in order to help those who need it most. "I have to remind myself that The Champion's Centre is not my business, but His," Klaas says. He explains that there are difficulties, but prayer and faith help him through, as does a belief that God has the solutions.

Klaas realized that people with a mental illness, brain injuries, or a developmental disability have nowhere to go if they are not sick enough to be hospitalized. Many of them are too sick to lead normal productive lives. The amount of subsidies that are given to mentally ill people is often not enough to pay for a healthy standard of living. "There is a real shortage of affordable housing, not to mention housing that can support people with a mental illness," Klaas says. "These people have nowhere to go except the street or be confined to a government institution, whether hospital or penitentiary."

Klaas did some research through the internet to find different group housing models. He was looking for a group housing project the could support more than four or five tenants at once and had a business embedded in the facility to help pay bills. To his surprise, there was very little that came even close to this concept. The building he had purchased was zoned commercial-residential, so a business within the facility was necessary to use the building for a group home.

Klaas and his brother Fred worked hard to bring the building up to code after purchasing it in 2001. Because his work experience mainly consisted of the grocery business, he faced a lot of challenges. Klaas did minor renovations on the centre by himself; it was hard work as he is not a carpenter.

"Often, I'd be stymied as to how to do something, like putting in a doorjamb, building an arch doorway or even drywall," he says. "I would literally pray and ask for the ability to do it. It wouldn't be long, and I would eventually figure it out." Later on, contractors were hired for the tougher renovations, to bring the building up to a finish. This was made possible by a grant from Canada Mortgage and Housing Corporation.

Other difficulties came when he had to approach the local churches, businessmen, social agencies, and individuals for support. It was a very humbling experience for Klaas, but he believed so strongly in the concept that he put down his pride and asked for the financial help he needed.

Klaas had always had the ability to reach people on an emotional level. He credits this gift to God. Many times, he would approach people to help his cause, and to his surprise they would write him a cheque. Several service clubs, churches, and businesses contributed large sums of money when asked to sponsor a room in the centre. Plaques with the names of the people have been placed outside of the rooms they sponsored. "The Dutch have a saying that basically means 'No, you already have.' What this is getting at is, if you don't ask, the answer is already 'no'. You may as well ask. I had to remind myself of this from time to time," Klaas remembers.

For the first year of the Ponoka centre's operation, Klaas was without a salary. He did not have money to bring home to his family, and did not have another job to secure an income. Joanne was working as a full-time teacher at the Christian school so they were able to make ends meet.

While working on re-modeling the centre, Klaas encountered challenges he had never faced before. To help overcome the obstacles, Klaas turned to God. "In dealing with new challenges, especially those that I have no idea how to handle. I take them to God. Inevitably, the solutions come."

Aside from his duties with The Champion's Centre, Klaas and his wife Joanne, provided a home for foster children. They have been foster parents from time to time since the early eighties. They take on the responsibility of raising these children until they are 18 years of age.

Klaas' struggle with restlessness and depression no longer affects his life negatively. It helps him to have a clear focus for his energies—a mission that is far from complete. Since beginning work on The Champion's Centre, he feels no need to pursue anything else. "The struggle is over. That doesn't mean to say that every day is glorious, our tenants that are the problem. It is the attitude, integrity, misunderstanding and complacency in Christians and others that are the most difficult things to handle. Many people just don't care. Those who say they do, often don't follow through with any action," Klaas explains. He feels there was never one defining moment where he knew what to do with his life. For Klaas, the Christian life is a worldview. He feels that he lives his life by the Word of God and that it is his duty to help disadvantaged people—the people that need God's Word most. Klaas has reached this point in his life because of his faith and trust in God's plan.

Klaas invested his time and money to build The Champion's Centre into what it is today. Despite difficulties and a lack of support at times, he worked to create a place that would house the mentally ill and those with developmental difficulties. For many, it was the only place they could go. The Champion's Centre's vision of helping those who need it most has come true and continues to come true with the opening of the Medicine Hat facility in June 2006. Klaas believes that this housing solution can benefit people in need all over Canada. With his drive and faith, there is a good possibility it will. Klaas' goal is to continue helping others and opening centres like the ones in Ponoka and Medicine Hat all over Canada. Even with so much work ahead of him, Klaas is committed and he is looking forward to what lies ahead.

"You MUST BE the change you WANT to See in The World"

—GHANDI

HISTORY

The Champion's Centre's growth has been more like the growth of a living than the growth of an organization. It was little more than an idea spawned from the desire to help those in need. From this simple genesis, the form of The Champion's Centre as it is today has taken shape. However, its purpose and goals have been changed and altered throughout its development. From very early on, it became apparent that those in need were most often in that position because of the lack of support for their individual needs. With this in mind, The Champion's Centre has strived to accommodate the needs of every tenant.

Klaas had previously desired to open up a drop-in centre where troubled teens could have a safe environment for an afternoon or even a couple of days. Unfortunately, this centre never became a reality due to lack of moral and economic support from the community. About five years later, Klaas and his wife, Joanne, were in the market for a revenue property. They were hoping Klaas' brother Fred could manage it, having recently retired from his marketing position with Levi Strauss. They came upon an old medical building in their hometown of Ponoka, Alberta.

"We passed a realtor's office and saw the medical building for sale," says

Klaas. "We decided to take a look at it because the price was right, never thinking that we would actually buy it. While we were looking at the building, I asked my wife what she thought the building could be used for, and she said a rooming house."

With Joanne's assessment in mind, Klaas began to look into it. "I began to research the need for this type of housing and discovered there was an enormous need. There was a real shortage of affordable housing, not to mention housing that would support people with a mental illness. At first, this was our target population since most of our tenants would come from the Alberta Hospital. After consulting with the Alberta Mental Health Board and before they became part of the David Thompson Health Region, I was informed that there would be operational funding if I were to open a supportive housing facility that would provide both room and board."

Klaas and Joanne strongly desired to provide for the disadvantaged, and with the promise of support for their endeavours, they made a move. "We made a ridiculous offer on the building and the four medical doctors that the building accepted it. That was September of 2001. The building had been on the market for a year and a half, and I guess they were anxious to sell."

Despite their good fortune in acquiring the building, Klaas and Joanne still had many obstacles to brave before The Champion's Centre would be operational. "I applied to Canada Mortgage and Housing Corporation under the Residential Rehabilitation Assistance Program soon after I bought the building. Six months after beginning clean up and renovations of the building, I still hadn't heard from CMHC. They had lost my file, so I had to re-apply." There were other funding issues that The Champion Centre also encountered. "In February of 2002 I decided to approach the Alberta Mental Health Board and ask what the process was to obtain the funding they had promised. In retrospect, I probably should have applied right away. I was told that no money was being given out for new initiatives since the whole medical system was being revamped. I was six months into the project, so I decided to keep on going,"

Without the funding he thought would be coming to support the centre, Klaas had to rely on his own resources. "He did everything by credit cards," said Klaas' brother Fred, who now manages The Champion's Centre in Ponoka on a full-time basis. "His cards were up to the limit with buying the place and renovating everything." Because the funds were limited, Klaas found himself having to do much of the work himself. Fred also helped with some of the renovations and he reflects on the work that he did: "the renovations were good, but if you really wanted to renovate it, you'd have to tear everything out, and that didn't happen here. We took a lot of the stuff out and painted the rooms. We did a lot of it ourselves." Still, their hard work and good intentions did not go completely unaided. "I had approached businesses and individuals to sponsor a room for $800 and fourteen people contributed even though there was no tax receipt forthcoming," says Klaas. At this point, The Champion's Centre was not yet registered as charity. "By this time," Klaas recalls, "My house was mortgaged to the hilt and I had Visa charges of $25,000. I was strapped. Fortunately, the Canada Mortgage and Housing Corporation funding came through." With this new funding, Contractors were hired to complete the major renovations and the whole building was brought up to code.

Although the building seemed the ideal location in which to house a relatively large number of tenants from a local population in need of affordable housing, it presented challenges beyond the renovations. "One of the problems we had to overcome was that since the building was zoned commercial-residential we had to have some type of business," explains Klaas. "Since both my brother and I have a love for antiques and collectibles we decided to go with an antique shop. We needed a place for our men to eat, so we decided that a public restaurant would also fit nicely into the picture."

The integration of business in The Champion's Centre provided numerous benefits many other housing project did not have. In addition to what the tenants pay in rent and the charitable donations the centre receives, the business helps to further offset the cost of running the centre. "In addition," says Klaas, "our homes provide the opportunity for the public to interact with our tenants through the businesses, as well as services. Our tenants feel part of the community, as opposed to 'there's the lazy house where all those weird people live.' Our concept offers an aspect of social enterprise. Because we have businesses, we are able to employ some of our tenants who are willing and able to work, even if it is just a few hours a week. Not to mention that we are an equal opportunity employer. We employ people with various disabilities. The Champion's Centre concept offers more than just a group home of men living together." Although it seems like an obvious model, few other organizations have tried it. "To my surprise," Klaas confesses, "there wasn't anything like The Champion's Centre in Canada and only something similar in the U.S."

With their unique idea and the renovated building, they were finally ready to reach out to people. The Champion's Centre began housing men on June 1st, 2002. It was not a smooth sail from this point on, there was a definite learning curve involved with running The Champion's Centre, both internally and externally.

The Champion's Centre has had to overcome many obstacles in its pursuit to help others overcome their adversities. "I thought I had the support of the community," says Klaas, "especially from the mental health professionals. What bothered me the most was, after we opened, support from the community dropped off. We were perceived as making money off the backs of the poor, due in part to former tenants that lived at the centre who spread bad reports, even though we had done them no wrong. Some of the professionals believed their stories and did not bother coming to us for our side of the story. This had some adverse effects, but the perception is finally starting to change due to the hard work of the staff and volunteers." With that said, the centre has already helped a lot of people—not only the tenants, but also the staff, volunteers and the community at large.

In the early morning several members of the community sit down to have breakfast in the café, they discuss the centre, and even the character the building itself seems to exude. "This used to be my old doctor's office," says Emberley Splett, a life resident of Ponoka and ex-volunteer at The Champion's Centre. "Where those guys are is where the nurses were stationed," she said pointing into the living area adjacent to the cafe. "Here's where all of the old waiting rooms were," she says while motioning around the café and antique shop, "It doesn't even slightly resemble a waiting room. The doctor's office was back there," she says motioning towards the tenants' suites, which were converted from the old examining rooms. Upstairs was a dentist's office that now serves as Fred Klooster's live-in manager's suite. "I think an older place has more character", says Fred. "And this isn't even that old, you know."

Built in 1955, The Medical Arts Building allowed for a number of medical professionals to work from the same building. This was an efficient means of conducting multiple medical practices, as well as centralizing medical services for the community. More recently the Alberta Historical Resources Foundation and the Alberta Main Street Programme have declared the site a historical building. A plaque on the front of the building reveals a bit about its striking style: "This characteristically post-war design dispenses with window frames and traditional ornamentation, offering instead an interplay of volumes and voids, and a tapestry of surface textures created by flat Roman' brick, fine raked mortar joints, and glass block window panels." It's a comforting thought that, even though the building no longer houses dentists and doctors, it still functions for the overall benefit of the community.

Despite the success achieved by The Champion's Centre, there are a number of things that both Klaas and Fred feel could have been done differently. Fred had expected the centre would be providing permanent housing for low-income independent-living adults, but now wonders if this was ever a realistic expectation on the part of The Champion's Centre. "I don't think it was," says Fred, "because we were expecting people from a mental hospital. But then what did I know, or my brother, even, about that sort of thing." Whether it was expected or not, The Champion's Centre needed to house individuals with various mental illnesses. Overall, this experience was critical for The Champion's Centre as an organization. It's allowed them to shift focus and better address the myriad of problems faced by all people who find themselves disadvantaged in some way. Danielle Klooster, The Champion's Centre National Board Chairperson and Klaas' sister-in-law, stresses the wide range of people the centre is looking to help. "They're actually just 'men with barriers.' Their barriers could be social, economic, problems with addictions, or mental illnesses. It could be any number of barriers they face. We have had residents at the centre with the barrier of addiction. It's kind of the chicken-egg thing. They may have some mental health issues, but was that as a result of the addiction? We're not there to assess that. If they are presented with barriers and they want to come live in the centre, we're happy to have them. It seems that our residents' barriers have largely been mental health issues and brain injury." Virgil Lawrence, the Chairperson of The Champion's Centre's Ponoka Board, makes a poignant statement about The Centre's necessity, regardless of any shortcomings it may have had. "Because the Alberta Hospital is in Ponoka, it was a good place to start, there are people coming out of the institution who need a place to stay." Various individuals and staff members have recognized the necessity of The Champion's Centre and hope that there will be other self-sufficient organizations like it.

In addition to the unique idea and dedicated staff, the overall organizational structure of The Champion's Centre has also been key to its success. Even before Klaas had completed the Ponoka centre, he realized that there was a much greater need than the kind of housing The Champion's Centre planned to offer, and he knew he had to proliferate the idea as a concept. "I needed to form a charity to get funding and donations to help build centres across Canada. I began looking for individuals who might be interested in helping, people in the community who might want to come aboard. I found five and we began working on becoming our own charity. Believe it or not, the government lost this application, as well. When we discovered that, we immediately re-applied and we were registered as a national charity on September 4th, 2003." After that, The Champion's Centre's organizational structure has expanded. The organization has numerous boards throughout the province, a national focus, and communities throughout Western Canada have been engaged in discussion about The Champion's Centre concept. With a lot of hard work, and maybe just a little bit of luck, The Champion's Centre will continue to expand and help people in need.

"'Tis not ENOUGH TO help the feeble UP, BUT TO SUPPORT THEM AFTER."

—WILLIAM SHAKESPEARE

PONOKA STAFF

Hardworking and dedicated people are necessary to run a non-profit organization. These people must be willing to work a lot, and for very little money. Most important of all, these employees have to care for the cause and everybody at the centre. It's tough to find hardworking and reliable people. It's even more difficult when you're dealing with the mentally ill. It's not an easy job to cook and clean for tenants. Some of the men living at the centre can't take care of themselves, let alone dress themselves. They need a lot of assistance. The Champion's Centre was fortunate to find such reliable staff members.

The staff at the Champion's Centre in Ponoka are all kind and accepting people. They are easygoing and understanding. It doesn't seem like they are caring for people who are mentally ill or disadvantaged; they are caring for their family. In 2006, the Ponoka staff consisted of Janet Stuart, the cook; Fred Klooster, the manager; Margaret Burnette; Tony Dewaal, and Sharon McGovern. Emberly Splett used to volunteer at the centre and she still stops by regularly to visit. The following is little bit about a few of the staff members.

Janet Stuart

Janet Stuart, cook at The Champion's Centre, is a people person: friendly, warm and caring. She jokes around with the tenants. She was born in Edmonton and lived on a farm with her adopted family for almost 15 years. She worked at the Co-op in Ponoka for about fourteen years prior to working at The Champion's Centre. "This is my cooking job. I managed a deli before, but this is quite a bit different." Janet says.

Janet's most relevant job experience to her role as cook at the Ponoka location was perhaps at the Alberta Hospital. "There are so many different walks of life there; starting here didn't really surprise me. I do like it here better though. I've gotten to know each of the guys' unique quirks." Even though she was used to being around people with addictions and mental illnesses, she still couldn't compare the centre to the hospital. "It's an institution there, here, it's like an extended family. But, just like any family, there are members who don't want to do their chores."

Janet always speaks very warmly of the people staying at the centre. "We have a lot of good laughs around here. They're a pretty good bunch. One of the guys bought me a little portrait of pigs from the stampede. The first week I was here, there were two fellows that got me a bouquet of flowers for Mother's Day." Not only does she care for the people at the centre, but the people at the centre also care for her. "There's such an astigmatism. People just don't realize. I used to be that way before I started; then you get to know everybody, and you realize that they're a good bunch." Janet loves the centre, and she wishes for everyone to be seen for who they are.

Homelessness isn't seen as a problem in smaller towns. Most people think it's a 'big city' problem. Janet has lived in both big cities and small towns. She relates her time in Ponoka to her time in Red Deer: "You always see people walking the street. I think it's a problem wherever. The only reason people don't think it's a problem here is because it's easier to close your eyes to 12 people than it is 1200." Janet stresses the need for more centres. "If The Champion's Centre wasn't open, these people would be at the hospital or out on the street. They're very lucky to have a place like this and people that care about them." Homelessess is everywhere, it isn't an issue just in certain areas.

Janet plans to be at the centre for a long time. "I told Fred he couldn't retire until I do." They have a light-hearted relationship. "We get along pretty well. He can be a great boss. But he gets tired too, you know? We all get stressed out. We're both due for a holiday. We're having a terrible time finding staff." Despite the problems, Janet is a believer in 'what goes around comes around'. By putting in effort and care into the centre, Janet believes that the centre will continue to be a success and grow.

Emberly Splett

Emberly has lived in Ponoka almost all her life. She moved in next door to the Champion's Centre in 2005 with her husband, Michael, and her cat, Mocha, and they've lived there ever since. She was familiar with the building itself from before it became the centre. It was her old doctor's office.

The existing cultural stigmas of homelessness didn't bother her at all. She knew about The Champion's Centre from the newspaper and she had no problem with moving in next door. "This place has helped everybody. It's helped me get to know all the different people here." She enjoys living next to a vibrant community of individuals.

Emberly started volunteering at the centre right away. "I guess God sent me here to help out." She helped out in all areas, "I would answer phones, cook, clean, and look after the guys." She cares deeply for everyone at the centre and worries that the government isn't helping out enough.

Her favourite thing about the building itself, aside from the fact that it's no longer a doctor's office, are the "artifacts" for sale all over the walls. The only thing not for sale the charcoal rendering of Jesus in the main room with a gold plaque underneath that says "The Champion". Emberly adds, "You can't sell Jesus."

She gets along with everybody at the centre, and although she doesn't volunteer there anymore, Emberly still frequents the place.

Emberly says that she would like to see more centres all across Canada. "The Champion's Centre is the best place to have. I hope it stays here for a very long time. If we didn't have this, where would these guys live? What would they do?"

Fred Klooster

Fred was born in the Netherlands and he and his family immigrated to Canada in 1951 when he was only ten years old. He originally moved to Edmonton, the weather was the first of many culture shocks Fred would endure. "I wasn't impressed. We got here in the middle of February. In those days, winters were a lot more severe. My parents told me to call a taxi—I didn't even know what one was." Fred was a little disappointed when he got to school and found out that he had to take grade four again. "The teacher put me next to two Danish girls thinking we could speak the same language. Danish and Dutch are not the same thing. We talked to each other—we just couldn't understand it." The cultural ignorance of his teacher's and the weather was only a few of his disappointments

Fred had to get used to helping out others at an early age. "I come from a family of nine. As the older sibling, I had to do a lot of the work. I even changed my brother Klaas' diapers and washed them. I still remind him of it today. He's now my boss." It can be tough to find a good compromise between work and family life. "Where do you draw the line? Generally speaking, though, we get along just fine." Fred feels very fortunate for being part of the family that he is part of. "We had a good upbringing, all nine of us did. It's a mixed bag here [at the centre].

Fred's business background has proved quite useful at the centre. "The marketing in my background helps me from a business standpoint. I don't think my brother has that, he is more of a visionary. Somebody has to have visions. But as far as business is concerned, I think I'm better than him at corporate things. Klaas' thoughts on the matter are always 'God will provide.' I do agree with him, but you still have to work at it. The money doesn't fall out of the sky. I think I manage the money quite well."

When the centre opened, there were some troubles in solidifying its purpose. Fred says: "This place was originally supposed to be for independent living adults. People who could take their own medication, know how to dress and eat, but wanted a communal setting and didn't have the funds to have their own apartment. For them, this would be an ideal place to be. We deviated from our original ideal and turned into a care facility.

Both Fred and Klaas learned very quickly that they had to adjust. Fred learned a lot. "Living in Toronto, we had a lot of people on the streets. But I didn't know what schizophrenia or bipolar were. I didn't know the different types of brain injuries. We've had a few of them here, and some are some here still. I've learned a lot from observing and talking to the Mental Health Department. There are tenants that have schizophrenia, some have bipolar, and some have both. People who are bipolar go up and down like a yo-yo. You have to be really careful until they are back down to their regular level. For one of the guys, that's been happening for forty years."

Fred wonders what the their tenants' lives would be like if only they'd received the proper medical attention. "A lot more can be done if it's caught early. If you don't do anything about it, you'll be on medication the rest of your life and without control." Many of these people have gotten to the point where their families can't deal with them. They have nowhere else to turn to. "One of the tenants has family living in Sherwood Park, Edmonton. They never come. The family just doesn't know how to deal with it, they don't want to learn about it either. They'd rather just stick him somewhere."

Fred sometimes takes on a fatherly role even though some of the tenants are almost his age. "There's one guy here who took drugs when he was younger and now he's like a child again. I call him a kid, he might as well be a kid. He's in his 50's. I think it's a good lesson for a lot of people that want to start taking drugs. He calls me 'dad' because his father can't take him. I handle his money too." Although Fred doesn't have any kids of his own, he handles the role quite well. "A lot of parents don't ask for help. If a child has a learning disability, there is help out there.

They just have to ask for it. Some people are too proud. Same goes for welfare." Fred suggests that, sometimes, pride gets in the way of raising a healthy family.

The Champion Centre has rules to uphold at the group home. Drugs and alcohol are not allowed. There are some people that have been banned from the centre because they caused trouble. "We had an artist here at one point. He did excellent portrait work. We would have set up an exhibition for him here, but the drink got to him. He's not here anymore." The centre enforces their rules strictly and there are no exceptions to tenants that break them.

Fred's position at The Champion's Centre requires much attention and he does not truly stop working. "I do enjoy it to an extent, but I can have it up to here. Since I live upstairs, it pretty much is a 24/7 job. People come knocking at any time throughout the night. I just need to get away, get a good holiday. By good holiday, I mean leaving the country. If I go to Calgary, I would still be thinking about the centre. It has been my biggest challenge. Last year, Klaas came up from Medicine Hat and relieved me for a couple of weeks, but I didn't go anywhere. I was still here for a part of the time, so I still had to work. It wasn't really a holiday. I would like an assistant manager, but that costs money. I'm not getting paid that well. If you hired a person in their 40's to work this job, they'd ask for 40 000 – 50 000 a year. I'm certainly not getting that. I would like to see more funding from the government, without strings attached. It may happen soon when the organization is bigger." It is important for the centre to receive proper funding and financial support. With it, the currently limited support system cannot grow and extend to help more people in need of it.

There are several other challenges of running an organization like The Champion's Centre. Aside from initial funding and community support, there are a lot of staffing concerns. "The challenge is mainly in finding the right employees for the job. Sure, a person can clean, but they should also feel like it's a type of mission. Not everybody has that; others are just there for the money, which is fine, but they are not as committed as somebody who is really into this type of work."

Another challenge is dealing with the medication. "I would like to have home care come in and give it out first hand. I'm not a nurse. When the hospital brings somebody here, that's the end of it. They might come in once or twice a week, but the money stays at the hospital. It costs between 600 and 950 dollars a day at the Alberta Hospital and only 20 dollars a day here. I think we should have our own care centre for people who need extra help." The solution for this problem doesn't seem too evident. "It's not going to be solved unless the Alberta Government, the Health Department or the Health Region get together and do something. In the Camrose area, they will go into private homes to give people their medication. This is a private home, but home care in this Health Region doesn't provide medication in private homes. There are certain types of home care that they will do, but only for a temporary time. I'd like to have somebody come in three or four times a day. A lot of the home care nurses are female and they don't want to deal with the men. That's another challenge." The centre doesn't have the money to hire a health-care worker. Despite a need for more funding, Fred promotes the concept before the organization. "We just need more housing centres that these people can call home. I think that's most important."

In terms of the organization itself, Fred's idea for growth is to start small." As the concept and interest grows, things happen. I know these centres are needed. There are a lot of kids who are doing crystal meth and things like that. They're going to have to be in centres like this. I think the concept is good—it just needs more public interest." More public awareness is needed. For example, the public doesn't think homelessness is a problem in smaller towns. "I think there is definitely a need. A lot of homeless people come from smaller towns. They'd like to go back there so they can be near their family but their towns don't have places like this."

The smaller the town, the less community support. "It's donations that we go by. Ponoka has 6 500 people. In a smaller centre, it might be tough to get donations. Still, it'd be nice to get a place like this everywhere." There are buildings for places like The Champion's Centre everywhere. "There are so many buildings available. Of course, renovating costs money. The Medicine Hat building got renovated, but it got the funding from different places in Medicine Hat. Medicine Hat has 60 000 people instead of 6 500. Maybe we could open up in the bigger places and branch out into smaller towns."

The Ponoka has had a lot of community support. "We get support from three of the main churches here: The Lutheran, The Christian Reform and the Alliance Church. But with the amount of churches here, we could have lot more. It's the same thing in Edmonton. There are a lot of Christian Reform Churches, Lutheran Churches, Roman Catholic churches." The church support and spiritual focus has gone a long way to help the tenants: "on Sundays, we have chapel service which is open to the public and the tenants. We don't force anyone to go—we don't force religion. It's mainly for people who are uncomfortable in a regular church setting. It's laid-back and comfortable. That's why it's called a chapel and not a church. It's basically an informal church service. "The spiritual aspect does a lot for the tenants. It's there if they want it. We plant the seed and God does the rest. They come to it sooner or later." The religious and non-religious alike are all pretty comfortable at we Centre. "A few lock their doors, some don't and some leave their doors open. It's a safe place. The guys have their own keys, so they are free to come and go as they please." There is both freedom and privacy in the group home. Having been a person who was particular about his personal privacy, Fred was surprised that he was able to adapt to a home with fifteen other people. "I can be quite picky about my friends and who I associate, with, but I eventually get along with everybody. We laugh together. I think that's a success."

Fred suggests the possibility that their increased independence is what helps them along. "Over at the hospital, they get everything done for them; here they have to tidy up, do their own laundry. They are learning, slowly. " A lot of progress has occurred because the tenants know that the centre is far more preferable than any of the alternatives. "Without this centre, they'd be on the street, or in the hospital. They could go to overnight shelters, especially in the winter. But that's not home. That's a place to eat and sleep, and then they're out on the street again. There are some places where homeless people can camp out and sleep in tents, Toronto and Red Deer have that. Besides that, there is no other place to go. It's unfortunate in a country as rich as this. It shouldn't even happen." Fred stressed the need for empathy. "Try living out in the streets for a month. No money and nowhere to sleep. I haven't done it, because I don't want to."

Centres are needed everywhere, every city needs one if not more than one. A small number of men in Ponoka and Medicine Hat now have a place to turn to. "I think these people here can rely on us. A lot of the people who move out want to move back in again, some of them do. The turnover is not very high here. It is quite stable, but I've got a waiting list. Other people have come in from out in the street and say, 'we should have something like this in our town.' I think it'd be nice to even have another centre here in town. So many people come here and say, 'do you know where I can go?' Women, especially. We need a women's shelter. I think there's a place in Wetaskiwin, a crisis shelter for women, but that's a different story altogether. There is a halfway house here, but that's just a stepping stone to something more permanent."

Fred can't find room for everybody. In year 2006, there were sixteen men staying at the centre. He said, "I have 16 guests and I don't think I'd be able to manage any more. If there were 30, I think there would be a lot of fighting. There are eight or nine on the waiting list now. I get calls from the Red Deer Hospital who've heard so many good things about this place." There are a lot of needs that can't be accommodated. "You can get wheelchair in here, but it's very difficult to move around. We don't really have the room for it. We had a person in here once in a wheelchair. He didn't last too long. I can't be putting the person's socks on everyday. He was only here for about a week. It wasn't fair for any of us."

How has Fred kept the place running so smoothly? Just like anybody, Fred gets tired too. "I haven't had a decent holiday since I started. I've asked different people if they want to run this place and they said 'No way! l don't know how you do it.' I don't know, either." Fred credits God, "Without God and Jesus, I couldn't possibly run this place." He tries to keep religion in his heart and an open mind in his head. "My motto is live and let live. I mean, I do what I want; they do what they want. We all have to accept who we all are."

In cases where one understands any of the issues surrounding either mental illness or homelessness, it's not very difficult for that person to see why the two crises are related. Unfortunately, both of these issues are often grossly misunderstood by the public at large. The homeless are able-bodied individuals who are simply too lazy to get a job. The mentally ill are imbalanced dangerous individuals who pose an imminent threat to themselves and society. Perhaps the melding of the misconceptions about people without homes and people with mental illnesses is the notion that, much like the homeless, the mentally ill are simply lazy: the mentally ill lack the necessary willpower to effectively cope with ordinary situations. Even though the last misconception would almost seem to imply a direct link between the two issues, all of these notions are categorically untrue.

"I *had* NOTICED that both IN the very POOR AND VERY *Rich* EXTREMES of SOCIETY the WERE OFTEN MAD ALLOWED to mingle FREELY."

—CHARLES BURKOWSKI

MENTAL
ILLNESS

Since urbanization several thousands of years ago, homelessness has been ever present. It has increased its presence with the rapid acceleration of urbanization associated with industrialization. Certainly, there is more than enough of Charles Dickens' works that paint a very bleak picture of an impoverished Victorian-era England. Homelessness can often be associated with extreme environmental and social factors. The fallout from the American Civil War Created rampant homelessness across the United States. Much of the poverty that plagues nations undergoing the process of industrialization is directly linked to labour issues. With the creation of employment opportunities, the ensuring of fair remuneration for a labourer's work can have a powerful effect on a society's economy. Although ideally this would relieve homelessness to some extent, unfortunately, it does not address reality. In any population, even nations with strong economies, there are those who are unable to capitalize on the opportunities available to them due to their inability to care for themselves.

Modern societies are constructed with support structures that are supposed to protect and nurture people in their times of need. However, many people take these support structures for granted. People operate on the assumption that everyone has family and friends that have both the desire and the ability to look after them if required. In Canada, people cling to the bastion of socialized medicine, it is the right of all Canadians—but it's becoming less and less of a reality. The truth is, despite the systems designed to protect people, there are individuals in the population that the systems fail to assist. When these individuals are at their weakest, the weaknesses of these systems are revealed. Stabilizing the social infrastructure in Canada, or any developed nation for that matter, isn't perfect. It's not unreasonable to assume that there will always be people the system fails to aid. Statistically speaking, the number of people who do slip through the system is relatively negligible.

In most developed nations, the number of homeless people is less than one or two percent. According to the United Nations Human Settlements Programme, the number of homeless people in the United States is 3.5 million, and 3 million for the European Union (*Homelessness*, 2006). In Canada, the National Homeless initiative admits that there are no reliable statistics on the number of people without homes (*NHI-reviewing the numbers*, 2003). This is a perplexing situation and can suggest a number of things. First of all, it can suggest social systems are working fairly well and that less than one or two percent represents an acceptable margin of error. The opposition will point out that in a nation of 30 million, one percent is still 300 000 homeless people. Paradoxically, the problem is both insignificant and insurmountable. One percent of the population does not raise serious concern, but 300 000 is a large group of people. The solution, it seems, is self-evident. Attitudes need to be changed.

There was a time, in the not too distant past, when large numbers of people suffering from mental illnesses were housed, often on a permanent basis, in institutions. These institutions were little more than a rudimentary solution to a problem that no one really understood or even grasped. While the institutions were not a great model for the promotion of mental well-being by current standards, at least they existed. However, many of the practices in these institutions were inhumane, even barbaric, and ultimately led to many people calling for change in the way the mentally ill were treated. Unfortunately, in many cases this simply meant the closure of mental institutions, and the patients that had previously occupied the institutions were released without adequate supervision or support. The release of occupants from institutions almost always leads to a rise in the prevalence of homelessness.

Those most at risk for becoming homeless are those who suffer from a disability. While it is worth noting that mental or physical disabilities can predispose an individual towards a lifestyle of homelessness, more often than not, mental disabilities are intimately interwoven with homelessness. Mental illness remains largely mysterious to the general populatio, though it is surprisingly ubiquitous. On average, one in five people will suffer from some sort of mental illness at some point in his or her lifetime. In 2003, the U.S. President's New Freedom Commission on Mental Health reported, "mental illnesses rank among illnesses that cause disability in the United States, Canada, and Western Europe" (*President's New Freedom Commission on MH: Report to the President: Executive Summary*, 2003, para. 13).

Mental illness is much more than just a disability that potentially places its victim at risk of becoming homeless. It wields a frighteningly power to destroy the lives of the people afflicted with it.

There are many different types of mental illnesses, all of which have variable degrees of severity. A mental illness manifests through one's own personality and it can be said that no mental illnesses are exactly alike because every individual is different. The American Psychiatric Association's Diagnostic and Statistical Manual of Mental Disorders, in its fourth edition, lists 17 different categories of mental illness, and 374 illnesses in total (*Mental Illness*, 2006). Some common illnesses, and ones which often place those who suffer from them at risk, include: schizophrenia, clinical depression, bipolar disorder, substance abuses and addictions and various developmental disabilities. The Schizophrenia Society of Alberta describes schizophrenia as "a mental disorder that impairs a person's ability to think clearly, manage his or emotions and relate to others" (*Information on Schizophrenia*, 2004).

Like many mental illnesses, schizophrenia is rarely characterized by only one or two symptoms. It is a complex condition that may present itself in a variety of ways.

There are general symptoms that are broken down into the categories of positive and negative. Symptoms categorized as positive, represent an addition to an individual's mental state of being. While other symptoms, categorized as negative, are a loss to an individual's mental state of being. Positive symptoms reflect the gain of mental functions and behavioural traits that an individual did not previously possess before being afflicted with schizophrenia. Hallucinations and/or delusions are perhaps the most quintessential example of a positive symptom. Auditory hallucinations are especially common. The voices associated with schizophrenia often appear convincingly real and are perceived to be real by the victim. Although an individual with schizophrenia may hear multiple voices, schizophrenia should not be confused with Dissociative Identity Disorder, which is commonly referred to as Multiple Personality Disorder. Negative symptoms reflect the loss of mental functions and behavioural traits that an individual previously possessed before being afflicted with or that might normally be possessed by an individual not afflicted with schizophrenia. For example, a person with schizophrenia may have trouble coherently organizing his or her thoughts and behaviours. In a conversational situation, he or she may repeat themselves excessively, or be unable to respond. In severe cases, schizophrenia may compromise an individual's ability to perform tasks most people would regard as routine, such as dressing oneself. The individual with 'negative' symptoms may become emotionally distant or withdrawn, perhaps even catatonic. Postive and negative symptoms may simultaneously manifest with any one victim of schizophrenia.

There are many theories on the causes of schizophrenia, a number of which appear to hold varying degrees of validity. Most theories only gravitate towards a chemical imbalance as being a major factor in the development of schizophrenia. It should be noted that a good deal of progress has been made through the use of a wide variety of medications, which usually offset the effects of hallucinations and delusions. It is a widely held belief that one of the most important things an individual can do in the course of treating schizophrenia to ensure that they are regularly medicated. This is often easier said than done, some individuals may require a certain amount of direction or assistance with their medication.

Schizophrenia has long been regarded as a heritable disease and there is now a good deal of evidence that suggests there is a genetic predisposition towards the development of schizophrenia. Despite that, it does not completely rule out environmental factors as potential precursors to schizophrenia. For instance, heavy drug use may contribute to the onset of schizophrenia. Although it is thought that for this to occur an individual, they must already be predisposed to developing schizophrenia. In all likelihood, it is a combination of multiple factors that lead to the development of the disease.

Clinical Depression, a more common mental illness, is probably one of the most misunderstood. All people experience sadness. The human spectrum of emotion is designed for human beings to be able to feel sadness. There are usually points in the lives of any individual where he or she will experience intense sadness, which is often referred to as 'regular' depression. Clinical Depression is different. It is a medical condition that is not completely explained. It occurs in disproportionately to events in an individual's life that might normally trigger such emotions. It often causes intense sadness for no tangible reason and will experience it more intensely than normal. Often, people will blame themselves for their condition. However, to an outside observer, the depression and subsequent actions—or perhaps inaction of the depressed individual appear wholly irrational.

There are a number of symptoms of clinical depression. Perhaps one of the most important things differentiating a clinical depression from sadness is the degree to which an individual is affected by the symptoms. Clinical depression almost always causes a significant, or at least noticeable, disruption in an individual's daily routine. Depressing thoughts take over an individual's mind until those thoughts dominate his or her daily routine.

There is strong evidence to support the theory that depression is caused by a chemical imbalance in the brain. Furthermore, depression seems to be a heritable disease, and people with a family history of depression are more likely to be genetically predisposed to experiencing depression. Circumstances and events such as the death of a loved one or the end of a relationship may trigger depressive episodes. Fortunately, as much as negative events and actions can have a negative effect on the mood and mindset of one suffering from depression, positive events and actions can have a positive effect on an individual's mood and mindset. Simple activities like meditation and physical exercise can play an important role in the management of depression. In addition, there are a number of different medications that have also proven effective in battling depression. While some people may find they do not require medication, it may prove necessary for others.

One of the most important aspects of effective management of depression is the identification and acceptance of it. It can be of great help and comfort for an individual to understand that there is a cause and explanation for the irrational feelings of despair he or she is experiencing. It helps a great deal if friends and family are also able to accept this condition and the person afflicted with it.

There is no real cure for depression, but there are ways of managing the illness. Throughout one's life, clinical depression will often fluctuate in levels of severity. On the one hand, there may be times when one requires a heavier regimen of medication, perhaps in terms of both dosage and types of medication, or even hospitalization. On the other hand, there will most likely be other times when an individual is able to function relatively normally.

Bipolar disorder, sometimes referred to as manic depression, is categorized as a mood disorder. Like schizophrenia, bipolar disorder is a complex illness that may manifest itself through a variety of symptoms. The symptoms may present itself in different combinations from case to case with varying degrees of intensity. At its most severest, bipolar disorder can be an extraordinarily debilitating condition, while milder forms may be much more manageable. The nature of the illness also makes it such that a person with bipolar disorder will likely experience fluctuating degrees of symptoms throughout his or her lifetime. The simplest way to understand bipolar disorder is to understand it as a shift mood within an individual between two states referred to as depression and mania. These states can also be thought of as 'lows' and 'highs'.

The depression involved in bipolar disorder is remarkably similar to clinical depression. There is little, if anything, to differentiate the depressive aspect of bipolar disorder from clinical depression. In fact, in the conflict of discussing bipolar disorder, clinical depression may be referred to as unipolar depression. It's been suggested that the depressive effects associated with bipolar disorder may be more severe than those associated with clinical depression. It has also been suggested that this could be the result of the dramatic swings between mania and depression.

The manic symptoms are what differentiates bipolar disorder from clinical depression. Manic symptoms are associated with a mood. It may include things like hyperactivity, irritability, hypersexuality, inability to sleep, and an accelerated, perhaps even uncontrollable, thought process. These symptoms have varying intensities. When they present in more manageable capacities they are referred to as hypomania. Manic symptoms are severe enough that a diagnosis of bipolar disorder can be made without depressive symptoms being present.

The bipolar disorder is more about the relationship between the various symptoms than the individual symptoms. While manic or hypomanic symptoms are likely to be the best indicators of bipolar disorder, the vast majority of people who experience manic symptoms also experience depressive symptoms at a much greater frequency than manic symptoms. The relationship between the two sets of symptoms is most often cyclical, with one presenting after the other, this cycle can even become predictable to a certain degree. While most fluctuations involve long stretches of time, some people do fluctuate on a more frequent basis. No one can truly be cured of bipolar disorder. Medication is prescribed in an effort to help stabilize an individual's moods and to make the symptoms of bipolar disorder and the fluctuations between them less intense. In this way, the illness is seen as being more manageable. Many people living with bipolar disorder are able to live rich and full lives despite the persistence of symptoms in some capacity.

The term 'addiction' is very broad. Medically, an addiction describes a body's dependence on a consumable substance that alters brain function in some way for a period of time. This kind of physical dependence on a substance can occur not only with the recreational use or abuse of substances, such as alcohol or heroin, but also the prescribed dosage of medication. Notable examples include painkillers or sleep-aids. In addition to physical dependence, an addiction can also take the form of a psychological dependence wherein a behaviour or usage of a substance—perhaps one that offers little to no possibility of developing a physical dependence becomes habitual. Psychological dependences are often implicated in addictions to behaviours such as gambling or sex. It should be noted that there is also evidence to suggest the internal production of certain compounds by the body while one is engaging in these activities plays a role in the addiction. While physical and psychological dependences can be described and understood separately, it should be noted that they often occur concurrently and ultimately produce more-or-less the same effect.

Substance abuse and addictions can have devastating consequences. Not only mental and physical repercussions, but also social and economic. Like many disorders that have province in the realm of mental illness, there is much debate surrounding how substance abuse and/or addiction contributes to a mentally illness. There are multiple theories regarding this issue, but there is no universal consensus on them. The physiological aspect of substance abuse aside, addictions of any kind can cause drastic changes in an individual's behaviour and cause major shifts in an individual's priorities. The chances are that almost everyone knows someone with an addiction in one form or another. The existence and persistence of these addictions may be liable to genetic predisposition to cultural landscape.

With almost any addiction, the pursuit of the addictive focal point, be it the consumption of a substance or the performance of an action, becomes an addict's number one priority. It becomes a priority that surpasses basics needs such as food and water. With addiction as a distraction, a person's focus on work, friends, and family decreases. This leads to distancing an individual from their support network and makes recovery more difficult.

The road to recovery is different for each individual; it depends on various factors. In cases involving physical dependence on a substance, such as a heroin addiction, a medically supervised detoxification program might be in order. It is common for medical treatments to be accompanied by behaviour therapy, which may include counselling or a larger support group similar to alcoholics or narcotics anonymous. Even after recovering from an addiction, the addictive urges may be present in an individual for the rest of their lives.

A developmental disability may be any number of mental or physical disabilities that occur early in an individual's life. Developmental disabilities may include cerebral palsy, mental retardation, autism, Down syndrome, and fetal alcohol syndrome. Although there is controversy surrounding the categorization of developmental disabilities, they are still medically associated with mental illness and the criterion for diagnosis appears in the Diagnostic and Statistical Manual of Mental Disorders (*Mental Illness*, 2006). In addition, other mental illnesses have a tendency to occur with greater frequency among people with developmental disabilities, as opposed to people without, although there is no single explanation for the increased prevalence of mental illness within this population. While there is a strong argument that developmental disabilities are fundamentally different than most other mental illnesses, there are many similarities between the conditions.

There are a number of problems that arise from a lack of communications skills or lack of social understanding. Developmentally disabled individuals may experience other health problems not directly related to their disability, but they may experience difficulties in communicating or health complications. This can prevent them from receiving adequate treatment. In addition, a severe developmental disability can impair an individual's ability to care for his or herself, compromising hygiene and health. Likewise, this can also happen with many severe mental illnesses. Even though individuals may have the capacity and ability to care for themselves, it may no longer appear to them as a productive or necessary activity. Unlike many mental illnesses, there may be no course of medical treatment for a developmental disability. While symptoms of schizophrenia and bipolar disorder may be managed with medication, it cannot improve the condition of an individual with Down syndrome.

Mental illnesses are extraordinarily complex problem and are classified as multi-factorial illnesses. They are conditions that are generally caused by multiple genetic and environmental factors. It can be difficult to understand for people who have not experienced it personally, but it is often even more difficult for those who are unfortunate enough to experience it.

While it may be simplistic and naïve to suggest that love and understanding can help treat mental illnesses, an increased level of caring and awareness on the part of the general public can only benefit. It is impossible to eradicate mental illnesses, but it is possible to reduce homelessness.

"home is A NOTION *that* ONLY NATIONS *of* THE homeless FULLY *appreciate* & *the* uprooted only comprehend."

—WALLACE STEGNER

TENANTS

While shelter is universally recognized as a critical necessity of life, a home is often very elusive and intangible. The physical necessities of life are recognized to be oxygen, water, food, and shelter. Humans can only minutes deprived of oxygen, days deprived of water, and perhaps months deprived of food. Shelter's position on the list is a variable that has less immediate effects. But, even the mildest and most forgiving climates can be subject to severe weather. In harsher and more extreme climates, people constantly deal with the unbearable heat or cold, or both.

A home is a place to belong and it is a reality that many people live their entire lives without one. Since June 1st, 2002, more than a dozen people have had a home at The Champion's Centre in Ponoka, Alberta.

Harold Arneson began living at the centre in 2003. He recounts the circumstances under which he came to The Champion's Centre: "I was having medical problems. My eyesight deteriorated to the point that I had to look for facilities where I could become familiar with and associate with other people. So, I ended up here. It'll be two years and ten and a half months that I've been here. I like The Champion's Centre because I've moved around most of my life. Up until I was 16 years old,

I went to about 16 different schools. I was born in Wetaskiwin, and lived in Millet. I've lived in Vancouver. I've lived in Calgary. I've lived in Lethbridge. I lived in Lethbridge for forty years, but never in the same building in all those forty years. It's the longest I've lived anywhere of all my life, in The Champion's Centre. It's quite a comforting to say there is one place that you can live for two years and ten and a half months."

Don Riggs' extended absence from his own home in Drumheller, Alberta eventually resulted in the loss of it. Don was understandably upset as he recounted the occurrence, "I used to have my own home until my mom sold it, because I couldn't maintain the house. My mom couldn't keep the grass in the summertime and the snow in the winter, so she sold it. It was my own. It was all paid for and everything. It was my own house." Don offers some insight into his absence from his home. "I stayed at the hospital first. I was there for quite a while. I don't know how long I was there. My nerves were bothering me." Eventually, Don moved from Alberta Hospital to The Champion's Centre. "Well, I just thought I'd come down here and try it for a while. It wasn't a crowbar hotel. And my nerves were still kind of bothering me." Even though it doesn't quite feel like home for Don, he feels more comfortable than he did in the hospital. "The Champion's Centre is actually better because you can go on your own. It's okay, but I don't want to stay here the rest of my life."

Lloyd McKay, one of The Champion's Centre's original tenants, says he is at the centre 'for good'. Lloyd suffers from depression, but since he has begun to take medication regularly and his condition has become much easier to manage. "I lived in the hospital for a year, a whole year, until I finally decided to take this Effexor. I was going to have a hard time going down to the drug store and going over to see the doctor and going to the bank and stuff, but I started taking Effexor and I could do it easy. I could do all my important jobs just really easy. So, I got the right medication", he says. In addition to providing a stable environment in which Lloyd can manage his depression, The Champion's Centre also gives Lloyd a chance to pursue some recreational activities. such as enjoying movies and playing pool. He is thankful for the centre's spiritual focus, as he feels it's helped him and his family. "We prayed for my son, and about a week after we prayed for him he met his wife. They got married, and now they might have a kid next spring."

Robert Ebl, originally from Ekeville, Alberta, thinks that The Champion's Centre helps him to live better, especially the wide range of options presented to him by the centre. It has helped him manage his mental illness better. "I wanted a big place, so I came here. I moved here from the hospital, I was there for a while to rest up and to get medication properly for myself. It's the best place for me. It's unique." Robert has also found a path to both comfort as well as personal growth from the centre's spiritual focus. "I'm living more spiritual." says Robert, "which is better. It's made me more alert of others' needs and things like that. It's made me more alert of other people and how I can help them."

Vince Cattleman, like the other tenants, also spent time in the nearby Alberta Hospital. "I am a schizophrenic, and I get attacks sometimes." Vince enjoys the positive and stable environment of The Champion's Centre. In particular, Vince appreciates the delicious meals The Champion's Centre provides on a daily basis, as well as the help he gets with taking his medication at the prescribed intervals. "I'm taking my medication regularly, I don't see things anymore." One of Vince's most striking characteristics is his overall friendliness. He smiles as he thinks about his time at The Champion's Centre.

Wayne Fisher, another tenant who is schizophrenic, also has to cope with the voices that speak to him. "It's just like you and me talking together, but you can't see him. They were going on day and night. I wasn't all there, that's schizophrenia." The illness has been with Wayne for most of his life as he continued to live in a variety of environments, including Alberta Hospital. "I lived in Red Deer for about 4 years, at a group home. I had lots of fun there. Then I went back to the hospital, they found me a place called the halfway house. I stayed there for seven years." As a hardworking man by nature, Wayne has been able to work in the community since moving to The Champion's Centre. "I work at the clubhouse as a labourer. It's just right down by the park, by the railroad.

It's worthwhile. The House of the Rising Sun, it's called. You can find a lot of interesting stuff there. They recycle bottles and things at the bottle depot and get money for that." Wayne has found that working helps his schizophrenia. "For 20 years I worked for one guy every day for five dollars an hour. I was a groundskeeper at the Alberta Hospital. That's when I had the voices and I had to get the help and stuff. It started to get better mowing grass everyday. It was something to do. I'd mow grass in the summer and shovel snow in the winter. I'd do two or three hours of work there everyday. It helped, the voices stopped." One of the factos that aggravated Wayne's mental illness was substance abuse earlier in his life. "I went to Olds Senior High School. I was born and raised in Olds. I went Olds College when I was 19. I took a John Deere Apprenticeship Program. I got started on the liquor. I was drinking at about 17 to about 21. Pretty heavy. I got sick on the liquor and cigarettes." Wayne has since quit drinking and smoking, and, in conjunction with medication, it's helped him to better manage his schizophrenia. "It's pretty clear. I don't hear nothing, now." Wayne now has the time and money to pursue other recreational activities.

Substance abuse is often a recurring theme with The Champion's Centre's tenants, Edward Rabbit is no different. He struggled alcoholism for half of his life. "I was an alcoholic for a long time. I think about it. Think about how much changed my life, how much trouble it caused in my life, all my ups and downs in life. I was at the Alberta Hospital for a while, about a year. I was suicidal. It was mostly alcohol-related." Two years ago, Edward was presented with an opportunity to move into The Champion's Centre. "They asked me if I wanted to move in here, and I told them I wasn't sure what it was like. They explained it to me, and brought me down to check out the cafe. They asked me if I liked it, and I told them I did and I told them I would move in." Edward has found his life at The Champion's Centre to be a positive experience that has allowed him to face his substance abuse problem. "I like it. It's a good place to be. I think there should be more places like this opening up. It's nice here. It helps me out. It keeps me away from drinking. It keeps my mind off drinking. I've been sober for two years, now. I haven't had a drop of liquor in two years. I don't do drugs. I used to smoke a lot of pot, but since I moved in here I haven't touched none of it. I haven't done drugs in two years, now. Not once, ever since I moved in here." Edward humbly concedes that it was neither him nor the centre was responsible for his initial desire to overcome his addiction. With a Christian focus in his own life, Edward appreciates The Champion's Centre's Christian philosophy that much more. Even though Edward is comfortable at The Champion's Centre, and appreciative for the challenges the support network at the centre has helped him face, and will continue to help him face, he feels it's still missing something. In 2006, Edward thought about returning to the reserve, but was concerned that a move back to Hobbema would put him at risk for addiction relapse and possibility of falling into gang life and possibly falling prey to the violence associated with it. Although these are all potential dangers, Edward is confident that the faith he has gained while at The Champion's Centre will continue to support him and his family.

Paul Semple became a resident of the centre in 2006. He suffered a stroke that paralyzed the entire left side of his body. Paul was able to regain the ability to walk with the aid of a cane. "Do you remember on the radio, they were talking about Vioxx? It caused quite a few strokes in the United States. I was on that, and they figure that's why I had a stroke. But, they figure the crack had a lot to do with it. After I had my stroke, I got really depressed and I ended up going to Alberta hospital." Paul is eager to talk about his life before crack-cocaine and The Champion's Centre. "Wait 'til I tell you what I did for a job, you'll really flip out. I was a senior engineer for an oil company. I built oil leases for Husky Oil. I'd hire all the contractors and oversee the job from start to finish. I had a lot of people look up to me, and I had a lot of people working for me. I just couldn't see my life the way it was. I had a Corvette and a 1970 Porsche 911 T." He was married for and has four children. Although he is no longer living with his family, they still keep in touch and contact each other weekly. Paul still had trouble living on his own after coming out of the hospital, He began inquiring about a place at The Champion's Centre. "I was living in Rocky Mountain House, on an acreage. I heard about The Champion's Centre from when I was in Alberta Hospital, and there's no place like it in Rocky. I phoned from there and got on the waiting list." Paul feels that The Champion's Centre has helped him with his drug addictions because of strict regulations. In addition to that, he has gained a home and a family. He plans to live at the centre until he is well enough to move back to Rock and work again.

Paul's addiction crept into his life and dominated it; he began to skip work. The oil company was concerned for Paul because his position was important enough to shut a job down when he was absent. He hid it from most of his coworkers and friends, but when he decided to confide in a coworker it became known to everyone. After losing his job and home, he had to live in cheap and 'shady' hotels as Paul put it, but he never had to live on the street. Paul says, "Cocaine is a terrible addiction. It's a pretty bad drug. It's probably one of the worst. I never stole for it, but I sold a lot of things that meant a lot to me. It's still a problem in my life. I didn't think, for a while, that I could survive without it." As much as he struggles with it, he has managed to become independent from cocaine. Paul continues to try fight against the cravings he still has every now and then, but he knows that it is possible to be drug-free through determination and conviction. He has a positive outlook and hopes to own another Corvette sometime in the future.

People who have experienced and know of The Champion's Centre's work and success hope to introduce the concept everywhere. Everyone at the centre believes it's an idea that needs to expand further and faster than it already is. There's a prevailing belief that what makes The Champion's Centre special is the philosophy of accepting anyone in need. This creates a unique and diverse home environment. The individuals living at The Champion's centre fit together and support another. When the right resources are put together in the right way, a shelter can be made.

"**OVERCOMING** poverty is NOT a TASK OF *charity* BUT it IS *an* ACT OF **JUSTICE**."

—NELSON MANDELA

MEDICINE HAT

On June 21, 2006, The Champion's Centre celebrated the grand opening of the Medicine Hat facility; the organization's second supportive housing initiative. Many of the people who helped with the Ponoka location were present to witness the ribbon cutting by the mayor of Medicine Hat, Garth Valley.

The new facility houses twelve single men and employs eight staff members to help care for and support the tenants and help run the antiques shop and cafe. Many of the tenants there are referrals from agencies in the community and from the Medicine Hat Hospital.

In 2005, Medicine Hat was a town of approximately 56 000 people located off the Trans-Canada Highway in the southeastern part of Alberta, Canada. Affectionately called "The Hat" by locals, the town thrived with jobs, houses and attractions due to its massive, underground natural gas reserves. In Medicine Hat, there are many without the ability to work and afford housing. Many people in Medicine Hat acknowledged this need and showed their support by attending the grand opening ceremony. The Centre officially began operating on June 29, 2006.

The embedded businesses provide work for those tenants who wish to interact with others and help sustain the centre. The Medicine Hat centre is home to two business initiatives that help contribute revenue to the organization. The money that the businesses bring in helps to subsidize the cost of housing a tenant each month. Tenants at the centre pay about $600, while the actual cost of room and board for one person is $900. The Medicine Hat location is able to function and be sustained through the café and antiques store, as well as thirty-five donations, funding, and fundraising.

The café that is run in The Champion's Centre's Medicine Hat location also participates in a hot lunch program in partnership with The Salvation Army. The idea was first put forth by the executive director of the Medicine Hat Community Housing Society. He approached Klaas about forming an agreement between The Salvation Army and The Champion's Centre.

The process to bring the Medicine Hat centre from a concept to fruition was very much the same process for the Ponoka centre. Klaas Klooster and his family were asked to come to Medicine Hat by the Executive Director of the Canadian Mental Health Association (CMHA) to discuss the possibility of opening a centre. After arriving, they gave presentations to the CMHA, the Health Region and some of the other agencies in the area, including the Crisis Assistance Network, a local group of 26 social agencies. The meetings were lengthy and took place over a few months. In October 2004, at the Champion's Centre National Board meeting, the board decided to relocate Klaas Klooster and his family to Medicine Hat to pursue a Champion's Centre facility there. To put the plan for a new centre in motion, The Wild Rose foundation offered The Champion's Centre a grant of $49 973 to hire both Volunteer Recruiter and a Program Coordinator for Ponoka. This grant also help account for the wage of the Executive Director in Medicine Hat.

During that year, Klaas and his family spent in Medicine Hat was filled with phone calls, meetings and presentations. A big lesson that Klaas learned from the creation of the Ponoka centre was the great importance of community support. "Starting out with the community behind the effort is a lot easier than going it alone," Klaas says. "Trying to get the community involved after the fact is a lot more difficult than laying the groundwork first."

Klaas worked hard to promote the centre and its benefits to every pastor and every agency in the community. There are chapel services tenants can attend for spiritual support. There is always a manager available to help with monitoring and administering medication, one-on-one tutoring, life skills training, assistance with finances, and social interaction outside and within the centre.

An important part of creating the centre was forming of a local board to help with fundraising, financing, and locating a building suitable for the new location. The people that formed the first Medicine Hat Committee and board of directors were: Frank Krulieki, Chairperson; Barry Roberts, Member; Lee Ann McDonell, Member; Gerhard Brost, Member; Norbert Klaiber, Member; Bob McGougan, Treasurer; and Brad Smith, Member.

The hard work of the board and committee was rewarded when the Medicine Hat Community Foundation asked The Champion's Centre to submit an application for funding. It was approved in December 2005, and the centre was granted $40 000. Other agencies took notice of the centre's growing momentum and offered their support. In January 2006, The Medicine Hat Community Housing Society granted The Champion's Centre $100 000, without the organization even having to apply for it. The centre received an anonymous donation of $50 000, and the Medicine Hat Board contacted them to offer yearly donations of $15 000 in 2006 and 2007. Through fundraising initiatives, the local board and committee was able to raise $13 000 through awareness campaigns in Medicine Hat.

With the fundraising and donations, The Champion's Centre was able to purchase a building to renovate for the new location in Medicine Hat, new furniture and professional kitchen equipment. The renovations cost about $107 000 to complete, the local board and committee members helped with the work.

Throughout the process, support was important to the success of the centre's start-up. From the beginning, The Champion's Centre Committee lent support through prayer, guidance and encouragement. At first, some of the churches in the community were reluctant to support the project. The number of projects that actually succeeded in completion were few that their reluctance was understandable. After a little time, churches in the community such as the River Park Church, Hillcrest Church, The Bridge, Medicine Hat Christian Reformed Church, and Victory Lutheran Church supported the centre through financial aid and prayer. Klaas believes other churches, which were not able to contribute financially, prayed and continue to pray for The Champion's Centre. "That is as important, if not more. When we pray. God answers. That is evident in the events that occurred to make the centre happen," Klaas explains.

"THE *sacred* formula OF POSITIVISM: LOVE AS PRINCIPLE, the ORDER as A FOUNDATION, and PROGRESS AS A GOAL."

—AUGUSTE COMTE

LIFE AT THE CENTRE

The only requirements for tenants are: low-income, cooperation with staff, respect for The Champion's Centre's Christian values, and willingness to share the facility with other tenants in common areas. There are rules are to promote a comfortable environment for all to live in.

The Ponoka and Medicine Hat centres require their tenants to follow a set of rules is determined by the National Board:

1. There is zero-tolerance for smoking in areas other than Recreation Room. A first offense will be met with an eviction.

2. Noise will be tolerated at any time, but more specifically between the hours of 10:00 pm and 8:00 am.

3. Tenants will be required to let the management know prior to departure if they are to be away from the centre for an extended period of time.

4. No friends or family may sleep over at the centre. If they are from outside of town, they are welcome to stay in an available unused room, if there is one. A modest fee of 35 dollars per day will be charged. There is a maximum stay of two days.

5. Illegal drugs and/or alcohol are not allowed on or near the premises. The tenant will receive a warning for first offense and will be evicted upon second.

6. Profanity and vulgarity will not be tolerated. It is a shared place.

7. Each tenant is responsible for their possessions. The Champion's Centre is not be responsible for any damaged or stolen property.

8. Keys are included in the damage deposit. If a key is lost, the tenant will be charged for its replacement.

9. Tenants' respective rooms must be kept clean and tidy to avoid infestations. Housekeeping will issue a 24 hour notice to the tenant if cleaning is needed. Management will charge a fee for the service if housekeeping is required to clean the room.

10. All tenants must clean up after themselves, especially in the shared areas, i.e. breakfast nook, shower and bathrooms, laundry room, etc.

11. A tenant must give a one-month notice prior to moving away from the centre. The room must be thoroughly cleaned. Any leftover deposit money after required cleaning and repairs will be refunded within 45 days from the move out date.

12. Tenants must take medication regularly by a doctor's orders if it is required to maintain health and well-being. If failing to administer medication(s) results in the tenant's hospitalization or other adverse affects, a warning will be issued. Second offense will result in eviction.

13. All new tenants are subject to a three-month probation period. In this time, tenants that do not comply with rules of the centre or has difficulty living with other tenants, management reserves the right to not to offer tenancy. A minimum two-week notice will be given if the tenant has not violated rule 5. If the tenant is disturbing the quality of life at the centre, 48 hours notice will be given to vacate the centre.

"We CAN no More DO without spirituality THAN *we can* DO WITHOUT food, shelter OR clothing."

—ERNEST HOLMES

LIFE AT A SHELTER

This chapter is in first-person; the information was gathered through an interview with a Western Canadian shelter employee.

Let me tell you a bit about the place where I work. It's an overnight shelter for intoxicated people. The facility hold just under a hundred clients. We have mats on the floor—no blankets, just somewhere safe to sleep.

We give them snacks when we can. When we do, they have a coffee before they sleep. We're pretty much the only place that offers this. Most places are open only at night, but here they can come in during the day to have a snack and social in a safe environment. However, in order to stay the night, they must be intoxicated.

We are called the drunk-tank; it's a place where the police drop drunk people off. It ranges from people who have been on the street for thirty years to people who got picked up after a hockey game. Sometimes youngsters are dropped off. They wake up, scared, with a hundred other people and no blanket. Clients are often bitter if we're at full capacity. They'll complain and say that we 'only let Indians in'. There's a lot of resentment about the situation that aboriginal people are in right now.

There are a lot of clients that come by regularly. They have day jobs to work, but they spend the night at the shelter. Many of the clients have issues with drugs and/or alcohol. Because there is a wide range of people staying here, trouble is not uncommon. Despite that, I love my job.

You have to realize how tough it can be sometimes. I mean, everyone is intoxicated at the shelter, of course there's going to be some animosity; people are always saying stupid things. It's very hectic around here because of that, especially in the summer. There are some calm nights and some that are far from it. Sometimes, someone will be snoring, another person will get mad and it escalates. There are a lot of guys with psychosis that worsens when they drink. We have to babysit them all night.

When it gets difficult, I don't get to sit down for an entire shift. Everyone wants a shower and everyone wants their laundry done. We provide both, but we can only do about twenty people's laundry in a night, it's too difficult to do clothing for a hundred people. There are a hundred people everywhere yelling, "I want my laundry done! How come he's getting his laundry done?" If we let the clients fold their own laundry, stuff always goes missing. They're intoxicated, so we don't really want them doing too much for themselves. Men and woman have separate bathrooms with one shower in each. Sometimes condoms are found in there. The people who have worked here for twenty years will tell you—this is a job where you'll never get bored. The overnight shelter is pretty crazy.

There is also a detox facility in our building. People are usually pretty grateful. It's for people that are really sick, prone to seizures, or people that come in with their faces broken in, which happens quite regularly. We operate with understanding that people aren't going to get help until they want it. If they're in detox or treatment, they have different chores to do. They have to clean up the common areas. But, because the organization is small, there isn't much to do. They're cooped up in this little area for detox; it's like jail. They have a bed of their own and a television they share with twenty-seven other people. They aren't in separate rooms, there are only small dividers between them. Some people walk out because they're bored, but we don't have the funding to keep them all entertained.

Most of our clients are 'career street-people', they just need three days with good nutrition and a couple days in a bed. Sometimes we let them stay a bit longer in our detox, otherwise they won't survive. It's too hard to live on a street for thirty years without having a few nights in a bed. When I say 'career street-people', I don't know how politically correct it is, but it's the term I use to describe people that have become good at living on the street. They are good at panhandling; they know where to get meals, and they know where to stay. Some of them have come from a long line of homelessness. Their parents, maybe even their parents' parents lived on the street. They grow up without a home, so it is normal for them. It's normal to get their laundry done only once or twice a month. I'm not judging or saying that they're bad; that's just what's expected of them and what they learn to expect of themselves. Some of them have street families, they form their own families and take care of each other.

Career street-people have become good at coping. I could probably never cope. It's harder for women. When you're a female addict on the street there are a couple options: become a prostitute, a drug dealer's girlfriend or... I don't even know if there's another option. I guess they can try and panhandle, but most of the time they are too vulnerable. They have to learn to adapt. They learn where to get meals every day and they have routines to follow. A lot of the people who stay here are here every day. It's like a career. It takes a very specific type of person to be able to survive on the street.

I think sometimes it has to do with their upbringing. Some never really got to be children. I don't know all of their backgrounds, but some of them talk to me. We have a lot of people that went to residential schools. I think a lot of them missed out on that family bond. There is a lot of pain and anguish in some of their faces. Then you get the people living on the street whose idea of fun is getting a bottle of Colt 45 and a handful of pills. That's what it's always been for them. I think a lot of them appreciate what we do—they appreciate attention. Not that they are all like "me, me, me," but they never really have people, you know, ask them what's going on. Lots of them stand on the corner and ask for change, or collect bottles all day. I think it means a lot to them for someone to just sit down with them and ask them about their day.

When people are hungry and tired, they're rough. I like to think, "If I were in their shoes, what would make me feel better?" A few quiet minutes usually helps. My main strategy when people are grumpy is to say, "Have something to eat and let me know what's happening." Sometimes people say nothing; sometimes people will have more going on. There was this one guy who came in and he was really quiet all night. He was hobbling around. Some guys were yelling at him, and he freaked out. This guy never freaks out. I asked him what was wrong and he told me he got stabbed. He lifted up his shirt and you could see that he tried to bandage it up with some garbage that he found. That's normal for some of them.

The staff are all different in dealing with our clients. I think it takes a certain type of person to do this work. I don't want sound high on myself, but workers are constantly being harassed. Some people just don't, and won't, ever like us. Staff have to deal with that all the time. Some are really good at dealing with schizophrenics and bipolars, others don't have the experience. We have schizophrenic clients we have to get to know.

There are three or four people that we just can't have here because their schizophrenia is so out of control. It's impossible to know when they're going to grab someone by the throat. Unfortunately, we can't handle those people. We have almost a hundred people. If we have three or four staff babysitting one person, we won't be taking care of the other clients.

There are a lot of guys that can be a handful but we let them in because they know us and they react well to a certain person who is working. Something that is common for one person will make the other go over the edge. We feel it out and work with it.

I don't know what the exact percentage is for people who have mental illnesses and are living on the street, but there is a correlation between the two. Staff working in the detox have to inform us if they have any conditions. There are a lot of people who need medication, but don't have a home or money. I'd say over 50% of the people in here at any given time have schizophrenia or bipolar. Schizophrenia is really prominent. They seem to like to medicate themselves and a lot of them are always drunk. A lot of schizophrenics try to use tobacco and intoxicants to regulate their schizophrenia. It seems to make the voices either more positive or less frequent. Drug-induced psychosis sometimes turns into a 'whether the chicken or the egg came first' debate. There's no way to really know.

We get a lot of people who come up to the door and don't know what our shelter is; they just want in. We'll ask them if they've been drinking or using and they say 'no', even though they obviously have been. They're so used to other shelters not letting them in for that. There have been young men, about 19 or so, that are schizophrenic. When we ask if they have been drinking and they will say they have even though they obviously haven't been. I usually let them in. Where else are they going to go? Someone who is schizophrenic is similar to someone who has been drinking or using. The same lowered inhibitions.

There are people trying to get in all the time. If someone says they've been drinking or using, there is no way to prove they haven't. Most people know that if they get drunk and picked up by the cops, they get in the front of the line. They'll wander into an intersection and get the cops' attention. They'll get right in—no line. Usually there is a line up for the first five hours we're open. When the clients come in they check their stuff, they get a pat down to make sure they don't have anything on them. But when the welfare cheques come out, we have lots of room. The week after, and for the rest of the month, we are full and have to turn people away.

Sometimes, we get referrals from other detoxing programs and we don't have the room. We work with other similar organizations and community organizations. Usually we try and take people out of the shelters-people will sleep there overnight and then come and use our detox. Those are the people we try to care to take care of the most.

The number of people we have to turn away changes depending on the season. In the summer, it's about fifteen people. People will come in for a snack and some sleep outside. In the wintertime, we have to turn away up to sixty people a night. Sometimes, I can't help but think, "If you sleep out there, you're probably going to die."

The government funds the shelter, but we aren't a government agency. Our wages and the building runs on the government funds but the food for people in detox and snacks are all donated. Most of it comes from the food bank.

We don't get paid exceptionally well, but it's a job. Sometimes there are days when I think, "What am I doing?" Those are nights when I wash 20 pairs of underwear people that were dope, people throw stuff at me and call me "white bitch." I sometimes I think, "Man, I was only there for four hours and I was called 100 names." But I realize if I don't show up, twenty-one people have to sleep out in the cold. We have a lot of troubles finding staff—we are always looking for people. The turnover is pretty high. It can be dangerous. Some people go on stress leaves after they get attacked. Sometimes, bigger organizations will steal people from us when they start to build up experience.

There are a lot of clients that don't use Assured Income for the Severely Handicapped (AISH) effectively. When they get their cheques, their friends come over. The people on AISH might have housing but, in the area, everybody knows who's on AISH. We have people who are in wheelchairs. They need their friends to help them get dressed. Often, their friends will show up, steal a couple of beers and then ditch the person in the wheelchair. Sometimes, they'll steal the wheelchair and pawn it off. They buy their friends with their AISH money. I understand that there is an important need for AISH, but there is also an important need for housing. We have people that get $1 500 a month and stay in our shelter. That gives people on AISH a bad name.

There are lots of people who use it really well, but there has to be a way of housing these people aside from giving them money. I know people need that type of independence, but there is so much of it that they use to feed their addiction as opposed to buying their medication—I see them going to the liquor store. Sometimes I just think, 'Wow. My tax dollars are paying for you to get drunk. My tax dollars don't pay for me to get drunk.' I think developing ways for people to be self-sustaining is more important. There will always be people who don't want to do anything. Either they are depressed or have other issues that they don't use what they're given responsibly.

Most of our clients are addiction cases. Usually, the people I see are people who lost their jobs or had a bad week, so they're drinking a lot. Three years later, they finally realize that they've drank their house away, their family has left, and they're sitting in a park downtown. I don't mean to over-simplify, but that's what it's like for a lot of them.

These displaced people can always find someone to hang out with downtown because they realize that they all have problems. They don't judge. If they have a beer, then they have a friend. It sounds really mean, but that's how camaraderie is. Once you get downtown, there is nobody telling you how low you've sunk. The family isn't there to remind them of how upset the kids are or what they have or haven't done. It feels alright to be out and be drinking all the time. But one day, many years later, there will be a rude awakening. I've had guys check into our detox and say, "It feels like I was at my kid's softball game yesterday." It's scary. It really could be anybody, especially in a society where drinking is accepted. Don't get me wrong, I go to the bar, but working here makes you realize how socially acceptable it is to drink all the time.

When I first started at the shelter, I couldn't drink. When I got off work and met some friends at a pub, I could not put the beer to my mouth. I'll never be able to use mouthwash again. I have people coming in and their breath smells like it. Sometimes they throw up; the combination of vomit and Listerine isn't good. When people use mouthwash, I can smell it. I cringe and they say, "What? I have fresh breath."

Working at a shelter has given me a different perspective. I can see some people can handle it better than others. It's a pretty fine line. I think about some of my friends who get dumped by their girlfriends and binge drink. I think, "What if your girlfriend dumped you, you lost your job and you got kicked out of your apartment all in the same week? Would that spiral into something bigger?" I won't assume, but it's scary to think about.

There are many clients, male and female, that drink to ease their shame and guilt. Many of them were once successful or lived very normal lives with families. We have some guys here that used to be really successful in the downtown community. They're disgusted with what they've become and don't like talking about their past because they don't want people to know how far they let themselves fall. Sometimes it's to the point that they need a drink or they will have a seizure. Some of these people have to check into our detox because they need a couple of days off. They have seizures all the time. There are women who tell us, "I never thought that I would be this bad." They have kids at home. They start thinking about their kids and they start feeling guilty. The guilt becomes so strong that they want to do anything to make it go away. They drink and end up hurting their kids more. It's the sickest sick you will ever see a human—they look like zombies. They are constantly dry heaving. Guilt has a lot to do with it.

We have some people that have been drinking so long one of his or her legs become gangrenous. They wake up and their leg is rotting off. Looking in the mirror, they see scars and all the things growing on their faces—they want to distract themselves. There are some people who are clean for five years and they fall off the wagon; they think that they've beaten it and don't need to go to meetings anymore. They get lonely and miss their friends, so they hang out downtown for an afternoon. It goes downhill from there. Having proper aftercare is important.

I've always been the type who can't say 'no' to people asking for change, especially in the winter. Even if they do spend it on booze, they're going to feel warmer. I always want to give them something. This job really opened my eyes to how many people on the streets have mental illness.

I was never really aware of that. I think I'm a little more cynical now because I've seen how people abuse the system.

There are many different things that lead up to homelessness: residential schools; lack of support for people with mental illness; people getting injured at work, they become depressed after being at home all day. There are people taking drugs from all walks of life. I started realizing what everyone's situation was; I realized that it wasn't just one group of people. People say it can happen to anyone and I don't really think much of it, but we have people staying here who were social workers. They used to do social work with the same people they now sleep next to. Former addiction counsellors now drink Listerine every day. You can see how addictions and other problems go right across the board. It makes me wonder what could happen to me years down the road.

Religion can help people. There are a lot of people who go to the Salvation Army and it puts them off. We have some people staying at the shelter who think they're Jesus. The twelve steps, it's based on the Bible. There is usually religious philosophy that is built into all the treatment centres. There are a lot of people who were in residential schools who I would have thought would be opposed to Christianity, but a lot of them wear crosses and say "God bless you." They tip their cross. A lot of them tell me, "Jesus don't judge me for sins, as long as I'm looking out for my brother while I'm down here." It's kind of surreal. Religion is powerful. It makes people feel safe. But, I think that's more in their survival than it is in their recovery.

Sometimes I wish we could do more. But unfortunately, there are always those people who push the limits when they see other people getting more. We have people that will mess their pants when they are standing in line to get their laundry done. They know how the system works. I just take it as it is. I'm not going to let it bother me. I feel bad when some people haven't had their clothes washed in two weeks. They're waiting patiently and then the same person craps their pants every day. It is frustrating, but we can only do so much.

It's kind of rare that we get to feed them because it's all donations. We try to give them a snack every night, but it's never anything healthy. It's usually, like, old doughnuts from Safeway. It sucks, but I do what I can. I always try to remind myself that even if I have a crappy day at on a twelve-hour shift on no sleep, I still get to go home to my own bed. That makes me feel pretty damn privileged.

Many of this country's citizens are unaware of the current situation. My father was totally blown away when he realized how many people from residential schools were homeless because they lost all ties with their families. He was amazed at how many people are homeless because of mental illness. When he found out, he said, "Well how could that happen? Isn't the government supposed to take care of them?" Homelessness is caused by the inadequacies in the current system and failures of the past. There isn't enough help to go around for everyone and the methods that are currently available to alleviate the situation aren't enough; money isn't always the solution.

"The INEVITABLE consequence of poverty is DEPENDENCE."

—SAMUEL JOHNSON

AFTERWORD

A person who is welcomed into a positive environment will be less disruptive and more respectful of others. Each person who calls the centre 'home' is given the opportunity to belong, and is offered help. The Christian attitudes held by the people who work with and support The Champion's Centre are the kind of attitudes we hope to see more often in our communities. The most effective way to bring these values into our neighbourhoods is to reflect them in ourselves.

We live in a society where it is more common to have a person brush roughly past another person on the street than say 'hello' to him or her. Each person we pass is not undeserving of our kindness; they may appreciate a smile and greeting more than we know. Instead of closing ourselves off, we should try to become aware of the plight of others.

One of The Champion's Centre's most important goals is to increase awareness of the problems facing many people at risk of becoming homeless. Instead of building a group home that separates tenants from society and society from tenants, the centre aims to integrate its residents into society. While it's important for the centre to participate in the community, it's also important for the community to participate in the centre. By opening The Champion's Centre to the public, much of the stigma associated with group housing and the individuals who occupy the housing can be stripped away.

That's why understanding and support of The Champion's Centre's goals is the next step. This book is an effort to convince readers that this organization is an effective way to help solve the problem of homelessness and the problems homeless people face. We hope that reality of the current situation of homelessness is convincing enough to bring forth the message that action is required and that the knowledge to take action is held within this book.

Where would The Champion's Centre be without community support? Nobody likes asking for something, but as Fred Klooster put it, "No, you already have". In other words, a person has to ask to receive. Help out The Champion's Centre—whether it is in your thoughts or prayers, with fiscal donations, with volunteer support or even just spreading the word about the centre. Your help could bring several people off the street or out of the hospital and into a permanent residence. Without it, some people might never be brought back into society.

The Champion's Centre believes, above all else, that everyone deserves a chance, and that everyone deserves help. But first, all of us must be conscious of issues affecting people in our communities. Only then can good be done to everyone.

"ONE FINGER cannot LIFT a pebble."

—AMERICAN INDIAN PROVERB

SPECIAL THANKS

National Board: Danielle Klooster (Chairperson), Zandrea Jensen (Treasurer), Virgil Lawrence, Austin Mardon (Public Awareness Committee) , Heather Miller (Public Awareness Committee), Frank Krulicki, Klaas Klooster

Ponoka Board: Virgil Lawrence (Chairman), Onno Roos*, Jean Avigne Glenda Eichler* (Secretary Treasurer)
*Previously on National Board

Medicine Hat Board: Frank Krulicki (Chairman), Bob McGougan (Treasurer), Norbert Klaiber, Gerhard Brost, Lee Ann McDonell, Klaas Klooster, Brad Smith

Edmonton Board: Christopher Holland, John MacDonald, Austin Mardon, Ken Nicol, Grahame Smith

Original Board (former members): Barry Roberts , Ernie Anderson, Jan Vaessen, Onno Roos, Peter Boodt, Bob Turkington

Ponoka Staff: Fred Klooster, Janet Stuart, Margaret Burnette, Tony

Dewaal, Sharon McGovern, Larry Davidson (former member)

Medicine Hat Staff: Helen Strugari (Centre Manager), Tammy Larson (volunteer)

Ponoka Churches and Organizations: Trinity Lutheran Church, Evangelical Lutheran Women, Sonrise, Christian Reformed Church, Ponoka Alliance Church, Parkland Reformed Church, Ponoka United Church, First Baptist Church Women's Group, St. Augustine's Church, Asker Lutheran Church, St. Mary's Anglican Church, Springs of Life Fellowship, Millet, ELKS, BPOE of Ponoka, Royal Purple Lodge

Medicine Hat Churches & Organizations: The Wild Rose Foundations, Canadian Mental Health Association, Medicine Hat Community Foundation, Medicine Hat Community Housing Society, Medicine Hat Real Estate Board, Salvation Army, River Park Church, Hillcrest Church, The Bridge, Medicine Hat Christian Reformed Church, Victory Lutheran Church

Various: Daniel Ireta, Staff at Service Canada, Archbishop Thomas Collins, Summer Career Placement Grant

And a special thanks to anyone else who has helped us out by visiting our centre, supporting us with donations and through prayer.

God bless you all.

For supplemental information:
    Visit our site: www.thechampionscentre.org

Toll Free Number: 1 (866) 777-7708
Email: champs54@telus.net

WORKS CITED

A Count of Homeless Persons in Edmonton. Edmonton Joint Planning committee on Housing. (2004, October). 2006, August 5. http://www.moresafehmes.net/HCReport2004.pdf

Calgary Homeless Foundation. (2006, November 7). November 25, 2006. www.calgaryhomeless.com

Desperation Rises for Families Living in Tents in Alta. Canoe Network (2006, September) November 25. http://cnews.canoe.ca/CNEWS/Canada/2006/09/24/1889468-cp.html

Economics of Homelessness. Parkdale Legal Organization. (2005, October). November 25, 2006. www.parkdaleleagal.org

End Child Poverty in Canada. Campaign 2000. (2006, July 4). July 12, 2006. http://www.campaign2000.ca

Factsheets. National Council on Welfare. (2004, May) August 13. http://www.ncwcnbes.net/htmdocument/principales/Factsheets_e.htm

Homelessness. Wikipedia, the Free Encyclopedia. (2006, July 13). July 22, 2006. http://en.wikipedia.org/wiki/Homelessness

Homelessness in Canada, Share International. (1999, April). July 25, 2006. http://www.share-international.org/archives/homeless-ness/hl-ch_Canada.htm

Housing Affordability Index. Royal Bank of Canada. (2006, September) November 25. http://www.rbc.com/economics/market/pdf/house.pdf

Housing Market Outlook, Edmonton, Canada. Canadian Mortgage and Housing Corporation. (2006, Fall). November 25, 2006. www.cmhc-schl.gc.ca

Information on Schizophrenia. In Schizophrenia Society of Alberta. (2004, January 10). July 23, 2006. http://www.schizophrenia.ab.ca/007-info/007-01.info.htm

LICO. Statistics Canada. (2006, May 30) August 13. www.statcan.ca

Mental Illness. Wikipedia, the Free Encyclopedia. (2006, July 16). July 22, 2006. http://en.wikipedia.org/wiki/Mental_illness

NHI - Reviewing the Numbers. In National Homelessness Initiative. (2003, July 3). July 22, 2006. http://www.homelessness.gc.ca/homelessness/h02_e.asp

Population. Statistics Canada. (2006, July 01). July 29, 2006. http://www.statcan.ca/english/edu/clock/population.htm

Presidents New Freedom Commission on MH: Report to the President: Executive Summary. President's New Freedom Commission on Mental Health. (2003). July 21, 2006. http://www.mentalhealth-commission.gov/reports/Finalreport/Fullreport.htm

Quick Facts. Toronto Shelter, Support & Housing Administration. (2006, June). August 13. http://www.toronto.ca/housing/pdf/quick-facts-2006.pdf